Tabl

Introduction

We are all busy people who don't have time to spend long hours in the kitchen cooking. Therefore, we all search for ways to make cooking easier. That's how many useful kitchen tools appeared.

One of these amazing tools is the air fryer. This innovative tool will make cooking so much fun for you. You don't need special cooking skills and you can forget about using so many pans, pots and different cooking methods. You need the best ingredients and you have to follow the directions. That's all it takes to make some amazing meals.

The air fryer cooks using the circulation of rapid hot air. This means you will always obtain perfectly crispy and succulent dishes in a matter of minutes. You can also use the air fryer to steam, roast, bake, grill and even sauté your foods. This appliance is sold with baking pans, grills and a basket to help you fry the food. An air fryer is worth having and it will change your cooking style for ever.

This brings us to the second part of our culinary journey. If you own an air fryer, you can use it to make some rich and delicious meals but not just any meals! Use it to make some fabulous Ketogenic dishes.

The Ketogenic diet is a high fat and low carb one which brings your body to a state of ketosis. This will lead to more ketones in your body but also to an increased metabolism and higher energy levels. The Ketogenic diet will show its benefits in only a few days and it will help you lose weight, feel healthy and look amazing.

Ketogenic meals are delicious and versatile because there are a lot of ingredients you are allowed to use. You can cook with greens like spinach, green beans, kale, bok choy or Brussels sprouts. You can also use broccoli, all kinds of cabbage and cauliflower. You can cook with fish, seafood, poultry, pork, lamb, beef, eggs, healthy fats, cheese, high fat dairy, ghee, butter, cheese, avocados, berries and plums but also with healthy oils like olive oil or coconut oil.

Make sure you don't use below ground veggies, grains, beans, almost all the fruits, sugar, honey, potatoes or yams.

Now it's time to start our special culinary journey. Enjoy the best and most delicious Ketogenic meals made in the ultimate cooking tool: the air fryer!

Have fun and enjoy cooking Ketogenic feasts with your air fryer!

Ketogenic Air Fryer Breakfast Recipes

Spinach and Eggs Mix
Prep time: 5 minutes | Cooking time: 20 minutes | Servings: 4

Ingredients:
- 1 tablespoon olive oil
- ½ teaspoon smoked paprika
- 12 eggs, whisked
- 3 cups baby spinach
- Salt and black pepper to the taste

Directions:
In a bowl, mix all the ingredients except the oil and whisk them well. Heat up your air fryer at 360 degrees F, add the oil, heat it up, add the eggs and spinach mix, cover, cook for 20 minutes, divide between plates and serve.

Nutrition: calories 220, fat 11, fiber 3, carbs 4, protein 6

Cheesy Turkey Bake
Prep time: 5 minutes | Cooking time: 25 minutes | Servings: 4

Ingredients:
- 1 turkey breast, skinless, boneless, cut into strips and browned
- 2 teaspoons olive oil
- 2 cups almond milk
- 2 cups cheddar cheese, shredded
- 2 eggs, whisked
- Salt and black pepper to the taste
- 1 tablespoon chives, chopped

Directions:
In a bowl, mix the eggs with milk, cheese, salt, pepper and the chives and whisk well. Preheat the air fryer at 330 degrees F, add the oil, heat it up, add the turkey pieces and spread them well. Add the eggs mixture, toss a bit and cook for 25 minutes. Serve right away for breakfast.

Nutrition: calories 244, fat 11, fiber 4, carbs 5, protein 7

Eggs and Bell Peppers
Prep time: 5 minutes | Cooking time: 20 minutes | Servings: 4

Ingredients:

- 1 red bell pepper, cut into strips
- 1 green bell pepper, cut into strips
- 1 orange bell pepper, cut into strips
- 4 eggs, whisked
- Salt and black pepper to the taste
- 2 tablespoons mozzarella, shredded
- Cooking spray

Directions:

In a bowl, mix the eggs with all the bell peppers, salt and pepper and toss. Preheat the air fryer at 350 degrees F, grease it with cooking spray, pour the eggs mixture, spread well, sprinkle the mozzarella on top and cook for 20 minutes. Divide between plates and serve for breakfast.

Nutrition: calories 229, fat 13, fiber 3, carbs 4, protein 7

Cauliflower Casserole
Prep time: 5 minutes | Cooking time: 20 minutes | Servings: 4

Ingredients:

- 2 cups cauliflower florets, separated
- 4 eggs, whisked
- 1 teaspoon sweet paprika
- 2 tablespoons butter, melted
- A pinch of salt and black pepper

Directions:

Heat up your air fryer at 320 degrees F, grease with the butter, add cauliflower florets on the bottom, then add eggs whisked with paprika, salt and pepper, toss and cook for 20 minutes. Divide between plates and serve for breakfast.

Nutrition: calories 240, fat 9, fiber 2, carbs 4, protein 8

Tomatoes and Eggs Mix
Prep time: 5 minutes | Cooking time: 25 minutes | Servings: 4

Ingredients:

- 2 tablespoons olive oil
- 30 ounces canned tomatoes, chopped
- ½ pound cheddar, shredded
- 2 tablespoons chives, chopped
- Salt and black pepper to the taste
- 6 eggs, whisked

Directions:

Add the oil to your air fryer, heat it up at 350 degrees F, add the tomatoes, eggs, salt and pepper and whisk. Also add the cheese on top and sprinkle the chives on top. Cook for 25 minutes, divide between plates and serve for breakfast.

Nutrition: calories 221, fat 8, fiber 3, carbs 4, protein 8

Creamy Almond and Cheese Mix
Prep time: 10 minutes | Cooking time: 20 minutes | Servings: 6

Ingredients:

- 1 cup almond milk
- Cooking spray
- 9 ounces cream cheese, soft
- 1 cup cheddar cheese, shredded
- 6 spring onions, chopped
- Salt and black pepper to the taste
- 6 eggs, whisked

Directions:

Heat up your air fryer with the oil at 350 degrees F and grease it with cooking spray. In a bowl, mix the eggs with the rest of the ingredients, whisk well, pour and spread into the air fryer and cook everything for 20 minutes. Divide everything between plates and serve.

Nutrition: calories 231, fat 11, fiber 3, carbs 5, protein 8

Herbed Eggs Mix

Prep time: 5 minutes | Cooking time: 20 minutes | Servings: 4

Ingredients:

- 10 eggs, whisked
- ½ cup cheddar, shredded
- 2 tablespoons parsley, chopped
- 2 tablespoons chives, chopped
- 2 tablespoons basil, chopped
- Cooking spray
- Salt and black pepper to the taste

Directions:

In a bowl, mix the eggs with all the ingredients except the cheese and the cooking spray and whisk well. Preheat the air fryer at 350 degrees F, grease it with the cooking spray, and pour the eggs mixture inside. Sprinkle the cheese on top and cook for 20 minutes. Divide everything between plates and serve.

Nutrition: calories 232, fat 12, fiber 4, carbs 5, protein 7

Olives Bake

Prep time: 5 minutes | Cooking time: 20 minutes | Servings: 4

Ingredients:

- 2 cups black olives, pitted and chopped
- 4 eggs, whisked
- ¼ teaspoon sweet paprika
- 1 tablespoon cilantro, chopped
- ½ cup cheddar, shredded
- A pinch of salt and black pepper
- Cooking spray

Directions:

In a bowl, mix the eggs with the olives and all the ingredients except the cooking spray and stir well. Heat up your air fryer at 350 degrees F, grease it with cooking spray, pour the olives and eggs mixture, spread and cook for 20 minutes. Divide between plates and serve for breakfast.

Nutrition: calories 240, fat 14, fiber 3, carbs 5, protein 8

Eggplant and Chives Spread

Prep time: 5 minutes | Cooking time: 20 minutes | Servings: 4

Ingredients:

- 3 eggplants
- Salt and black pepper to the taste
- 2 tablespoons chives, chopped
- 2 tablespoons olive oil
- 2 teaspoons sweet paprika

Directions:

Put the eggplants in your air fryer's basket and cook them for 20 minutes at 380 degrees F. Peel the eggplants, put them in a blender, add the rest of the ingredients, pulse well, divide into bowls and serve for breakfast.

Nutrition: calories 190, fat 7, fiber 3, carbs 5, protein 3

Cheesy Brussels Sprouts and Eggs

Prep time: 5 minutes | Cooking time: 20 minutes | Servings: 4

Ingredients:

- 1 tablespoon olive oil
- 1 pound Brussels sprouts, shredded
- 4 eggs, whisked
- ½ cup coconut cream
- Salt and black pepper to the taste
- 1 tablespoon chives, chopped
- ¼ cup cheddar cheese, shredded

Directions:

Preheat the Air Fryer at 360 degrees F and grease it with the oil. Spread the Brussels sprouts on the bottom of the fryer, then add the eggs mixed with the rest of the ingredients, toss a bit and cook for 20 minutes. Divide between plates and serve.

Nutrition: calories 242, fat 12, fiber 3, carbs 5, protein 9

Cheddar and Broccoli Bake
Prep time: 5 minutes | Cooking time: 25 minutes | Servings: 4

Ingredients:
- 1 broccoli head, florets separated and roughly chopped
- 2 ounces cheddar cheese, grated
- 4 eggs, whisked
- 1 cup almond milk
- 2 teaspoons cilantro, chopped
- Salt and black pepper to the taste

Directions:
In a bowl, mix the eggs with the milk, cilantro, salt and pepper and whisk. Put the broccoli in your air fryer, add the eggs mix over it, spread, sprinkle the cheese on top, cook at 350 degrees F for 25 minutes, divide between plates and serve for breakfast.

Nutrition: calories 214, fat 14, fiber 2, carbs 4, protein 9

Basil Mozzarella Eggs
Prep time: 5 minutes | Cooking time: 20 minutes | Servings: 4

Ingredients:
- 2 tablespoons butter, melted
- 6 teaspoons basil pesto
- 1 cup mozzarella cheese, grated
- 6 eggs, whisked
- 2 tablespoons basil, chopped
- A pinch of salt and black pepper

Directions:
In a bowl, mix all the ingredients except the butter and whisk them well. Preheat your Air Fryer at 360 degrees F, drizzle the butter on the bottom, spread the eggs mix, cook for 20 minutes and serve for breakfast.

Nutrition: calories 207, fat 14, fiber 3, carbs 4, protein 8

Cherry Tomatoes Omelet
Prep time: 5 minutes | Cooking time: 20 minutes | Servings: 4

Ingredients:

- 4 eggs, whisked
- 1 pound cherry tomatoes, halved
- 1 tablespoon parsley, chopped
- Cooking spray
- 1 tablespoon cheddar, grated
- Salt and black pepper to the taste

Directions:

Put the tomatoes in the air fryer's basket, cook at 360 degrees F for 5 minutes and transfer them to the baking pan that fits the machine greased with cooking spray. In a bowl, mix the eggs with the remaining ingredients, whisk, pour over the tomatoes an cook at 360 degrees F for 15 minutes. Serve right away for breakfast.

Nutrition: calories 230, fat 14, fiber 3, carbs 5, protein 11

Zucchini Spread
Prep time: 5 minutes | Cooking time: 15 minutes | Servings: 4

Ingredients:

- 4 zucchinis, roughly chopped
- 1 tablespoon sweet paprika
- Salt and black pepper to the taste
- 1 tablespoon butter, melted

Directions:

Grease a baking pan that fits the Air Fryer with the butter, add all the ingredients, toss, and cook at 360 degrees F for 15 minutes. Transfer to a blender, pulse well, divide into bowls and serve for breakfast.

Nutrition: calories 240, fat 14, fiber 2, carbs 5, protein 11

Parsley and Avocado Omelet
Prep time: 5 minute | Cooking time: 15 minutes | Servings: 4

Ingredients:

- 4 eggs, whisked
- 1 tablespoon parsley, chopped
- ½ teaspoons cheddar cheese, shredded
- 1 avocado, peeled, pitted and cubed
- Cooking spray

Directions:

In a bowl, mix all the ingredients except the cooking spray and whisk well. Grease a baking pan that fits the Air Fryer with the cooking spray, pour the omelet mix, spread, introduce the pan in the machine and cook at 370 degrees F for 15 minutes. Serve for breakfast.

Nutrition: calories 240, fat 13, fiber 4, carbs 6, protein 9

Creamy Spinach Spread
Prep time: 5 minutes | Cooking time: 10 minutes | Servings: 4

Ingredients:

- 2 tablespoons coconut cream
- 3 cups spinach leaves
- 2 tablespoons cilantro
- 2 tablespoons bacon, cooked and crumbled
- Salt and black pepper to the taste

Directions:

In a pan that fits the air fryer, combine all the ingredients except the bacon, put the pan in the machine and cook at 360 degrees F for 10 minutes. Transfer to a blender, pulse well, divide into bowls and serve with bacon sprinkled on top.

Nutrition: calories 200, fat 4, fiber 2, carbs 4, protein 4

Spinach and Eggplant Frittata
Prep time: 5 minutes | Cooking time: 20 minutes | Servings: 4

Ingredients:

- 1 tablespoon chives, chopped
- 1 eggplant, cubed
- 8 ounces spinach, torn
- Cooking spray
- 6 eggs, whisked
- Salt and black pepper to the taste

Directions:

In a bowl, mix the eggs with the rest of the ingredients except the cooking spray and whisk well. Grease a pan that fits your air fryer with the cooking spray, pour the frittata mix, spread and put the pan in the machine. Cook at 380 degrees F for 20 minutes, divide between plates and serve for breakfast.

Nutrition: calories 240, fat 8, fiber 3, carbs 6, protein 12

Cheesy Spinach Muffins
Prep time: 5 minutes | Cooking time: 15 minutes | Servings: 4

Ingredients:

- 2 eggs, whisked
- Cooking spray
- 1 and ½ cups coconut milk
- 1 tablespoon baking powder
- 4 ounces baby spinach, chopped
- 2 ounces parmesan cheese, grated
- 3 ounces almond flour

Directions:

In a bowl, mix all the ingredients except the cooking spray and whisk really well. Grease a muffin pan that fits your air fryer with the cooking spray, divide the muffins mix, introduce the pan in the air fryer, cook at 380 degrees F for 15 minutes, divide between plates and serve.

Nutrition: calories 210, fat 12, fiber 3, carbs 5, protein 8

Creamy Red Bell Peppers Salad
Prep time: 5 minutes | Cooking time: 20 minutes | Servings: 4

Ingredients:

- ½ cup cheddar cheese, shredded
- 2 tablespoons chives, chopped
- A pinch of salt and black pepper
- ¼ cup coconut cream
- 1 cup red bell peppers, chopped
- Cooking spray

Directions:

In a bowl, mix all the ingredients except the cooking spray and whisk well. Pour the mix in a baking pan that fits the air fryer greased with cooking spray and place the pan in the machine. Cook at 360 degrees F for 20 minutes, divide between plates and serve for breakfast.

Nutrition: calories 220, fat 14, fiber 2, carbs 5, protein 11

Kale and Eggplant Eggs
Prep time: 10 minutes | Cooking time: 20 minutes | Servings: 4

Ingredients:

- 1 eggplant, cubed
- 4 eggs, whisked
- 2 teaspoons cilantro, chopped
- Salt and black pepper to the taste
- ½ teaspoon Italian seasoning
- Cooking spray
- ½ cup kale, chopped
- 2 tablespoons cheddar, grated
- 2 tablespoons fresh basil, chopped

Directions:

In a bowl, mix all the ingredients except the cooking spray and whisk well. Grease a pan that fits your air fryer with the cooking spray, pour the eggs mix, spread, put the pan in the machine and cook at 370 degrees F for 20 minutes. Divide the mix between plates and serve for breakfast.

Nutrition: calories 241, fat 11, fiber 4, carbs 5, protein 12

Creamy Bell Peppers Bake
Prep time: 5 minutes | Cooking time: 30 minutes | Servings: 6

Ingredients:
- Cooking spray
- 2 cups green and red bell pepper, chopped
- 2 spring onions, chopped
- 1 teaspoon thyme, chopped
- Salt and black pepper to the taste
- 1 cup coconut cream
- 4 eggs, whisked
- 1 cup cheddar cheese, grated

Directions:
In a bowl, mix all the ingredients except the cooking spray and the cheese and whisk well. Grease a pan that fits the air fryer with the cooking spray, pour the bell peppers and eggs mixture, spread, sprinkle the cheese on top, put the pan in the machine and cook at 350 degrees F for 30 minutes. Divide between plates and serve for breakfast.

Nutrition: calories 251, fat 16, fiber 3, carbs 6, protein 11

Yogurt Omelet
Prep time: 5 minutes | Cooking time: 20 minutes | Servings: 4

Ingredients:
- Cooking spray
- Salt and black pepper to the taste
- 1 and ½ cups Greek yogurt
- 4 eggs, whisked
- 1 tablespoon chives, chopped
- 1 tablespoon cilantro, chopped

Directions:
In a bowl, mix all the ingredients except the cooking spray and whisk well. Grease a pan that fits the air fryer with the cooking spray, pour the eggs mix, spread well, put the pan into the machine and cook the omelet at 360 degrees F for 20 minutes. Divide between plates and serve for breakfast.

Nutrition: calories 221, fat 14, fiber 4, carbs 6, protein 11

Asparagus Salad
Prep time: 5 minutes | Cooking time: 10 minutes | Servings: 4

Ingredients:

- 1 bunch asparagus, trimmed
- 1 cup baby arugula
- 1 tablespoon cheddar cheese, grated
- 1 tablespoon balsamic vinegar
- A pinch of salt and black pepper
- Cooking spray

Directions:

Put the asparagus in your air fryer's basket, grease with cooking spray, season with salt and pepper and cook at 360 degrees F for 10 minutes. In a bowl, mix the asparagus with the arugula and the vinegar, toss, divide between plates and serve hot with cheese sprinkled on top.

Nutrition: calories 200, fat 5, fiber 1, carbs 4, protein 5

Green Beans and Tomatoes Salad
Prep time: 5 minutes | Cooking time: 20 minutes | Servings: 4

Ingredients:

- 2 cups green beans, cut into medium pieces
- 2 cups tomatoes, cubed
- Salt and black pepper to the taste
- 1 teaspoon hot paprika
- 1 tablespoons cilantro, chopped
- Cooking spray

Directions:

In a bowl, mix all the ingredients except the cooking spray and the cilantro and whisk them well. Grease a pan that fits the air fryer with the cooking spray, pour the green beans and tomatoes mix into the pan, sprinkle the cilantro on top, put the pan into the machine and cook at 360 degrees F for 20 minutes. Serve right away.

Nutrition: calories 222, fat 11, fiber 4, carbs 6, protein 12

Cilantro Omelet

Prep time: 5 minutes | Cooking time: 20 minutes | Servings: 4

Ingredients:

- 6 eggs, whisked
- 1 cup cilantro, chopped
- Cooking spray
- 1 cup mozzarella, shredded
- Salt and black pepper to the taste

Directions:

In a bowl, mix all the ingredients except the cooking spray and whisk well. Grease a pan that fits your air fryer with the cooking spray, pour the eggs mix, spread, put the pan into the machine and cook at 350 degrees F for 20 minutes. Divide the omelet between plates and serve for breakfast.

Nutrition: calories 270, fat 15, fiber 3, carbs 5, protein 9

Almond Chicken Bake

Prep time: 5 minutes | Cooking time: 25 minutes | Servings: 4

Ingredients:

- ¼ cup almonds, chopped
- ½ cup almond milk
- 4 eggs, whisked
- 1 cup chicken meat, cooked and shredded
- ½ teaspoon oregano, dried
- Cooking spray
- Salt and black pepper to the taste

Directions:

In a bowl, mix the eggs with the rest of the ingredients except the cooking spray and whisk well. Grease a baking pan with the cooking spray, pour the chicken mix into the pan, put the pan in the machine and cook the omelet at 350 degrees F for 25 minutes. Divide between plates and serve for breakfast.

Nutrition: calories 216, fat 11, fiber 3, carbs 5, protein 9

Coconut Cream and Avocado Bake

Prep time: 5 minutes | Cooking time: 20 minutes | Servings: 4

Ingredients:

- 2 eggs, whisked
- 1 tablespoon olive oil
- 1 avocado, pitted, peeled and cubed
- 2 spring onions, chopped
- Salt and black pepper to the taste
- 1 ounce parmesan cheese, grated
- ½ cup coconut cream

Directions:

In a bowl, mix the eggs with the rest of the ingredients except the oil and whisk well. Grease a baking pan that fits the air fryer with the oil, pour the avocado mix, spread, put the pan in the machine and cook at 360 degrees F for 20 minutes. Divide between plates and serve for breakfast.

Nutrition: calories 271, fat 14, fiber 3, carbs 5, protein 11

Olives and Kale Mix

Prep time: 5 minutes | Cooking time: 20 minutes | Servings: 4

Ingredients:

- ½ cup black olives, pitted and sliced
- 1 cup kale, chopped
- 2 tablespoons cheddar, grated
- 4 eggs, whisked
- Cooking spray
- A pinch of salt and black pepper

Directions:

In a bowl, mix the eggs with the rest of the ingredients except the cooking spray and whisk well. Grease a pan that fits the air fryer with the cooking spray, pour the olives mixture inside, spread, put the pan into the machine, and cook at 360 degrees F for 20 minutes. Serve for breakfast hot.

Nutrition: calories 220, fat 13, fiber 4, carbs 6, protein 12

Swiss Chard and Tomatoes Bake

Prep time: 5 *minutes* | *Cooking time:* 15 *minutes* | *Servings:* 4

Ingredients:

- 4 eggs, whisked
- 1 teaspoon olive oil
- 3 ounces Swiss chard, chopped
- 1 cup tomatoes, cubed
- Salt and black pepper to the taste

Directions:

In a bowl, mix the eggs with the rest of the ingredients except the oil and whisk well. Grease a pan that fits the fryer with the oil, pour the swish chard mix and cook at 359 degrees F for 15 minutes. Divide between plates and serve for breakfast.

Nutrition: calories 202, fat 14, fiber 3, carbs 5, protein 12

Salmon Eggs

Prep time: 5 *minutes* | *Cooking time:* 20 *minutes* | *Servings:* 4

Ingredients:

- A drizzle of olive oil
- 1 spring onion, chopped
- 1 cup smoked salmon, skinless, boneless and flaked
- 4 eggs, whisked
- A pinch of salt and black pepper
- ¼ cup baby spinach
- 4 tablespoon parmesan, grated

Directions:

In a bowl, mix the eggs with the rest of the ingredients except the oil and whisk well. Grease the Air Fryer with the oil, preheat it at 360 degrees F, pour the eggs and salmon mix and cook for 20 minutes. Divide between plates and serve for breakfast.

Nutrition: calories 230, fat 12, fiber 3, carbs 5, protein 12

Cheese and Mushrooms Spread
Prep time: 5 minutes | Cooking time: 20 minutes | Servings: 4

Ingredients:
- 1 cup white mushrooms
- ¼ cup mozzarella, shredded
- ½ cup coconut cream
- A pinch of salt and black pepper
- Cooking spray

Directions:
Put the mushrooms in your air fryer's basket, grease with cooking spray and cook at 370 degrees F for 20 minutes. Transfer to a blender, add the remaining ingredients, pulse well, divide into bowls and serve as a spread.

Nutrition: calories 202, fat 12, fiber 2, carbs 5, protein 7

Tuna and Spring Onions Salad
Prep time: 5 minutes | Cooking time: 15 minutes | Servings: 4

Ingredients:
- 14 ounces canned tuna, drained and flaked
- 1 cup arugula
- 2 spring onions, chopped
- 1 tablespoon olive oil
- A pinch of salt and black pepper

Directions:
In a bowl, all the ingredients except the oil and the arugula and whisk. Preheat the Air Fryer over 360 degrees F, add the oil and grease it. Pour the tuna mix, stir well, and cook for 15 minutes. In a salad bowl, combine the arugula with the tuna mix, toss and serve for breakfast.

Nutrition: calories 212, fat 8, fiber 3, carbs 5, protein 8

Minty Eggs
Prep time: 5 minutes | Cooking time: 8 minutes | Servings: 4

Ingredients:
- 1 tablespoon olive oil
- 1 and ½ cup coconut cream
- 8 eggs, whisked
- ½ cup mint, chopped
- Salt and black pepper to the taste

Directions:
In a bowl, mix the cream with salt, pepper, eggs and mint, whisk, pour into the air fryer greased with the oil, spread, cook at 350 degrees F for 8 minutes, divide between plates and serve.

Nutrition: calories 212, fat 9, fiber 4, carbs 5, protein 11

Coconut Oatmeal
Prep time: 5 minutes | Cooking time: 15 minutes | Servings: 4

Ingredients:
- 2 cups almond milk
- 1 cup coconut, shredded
- 2 teaspoons stevia
- 2 teaspoons vanilla extract

Directions:
In a pan that fits your air fryer, mix all the ingredients, stir well, introduce the pan in the machine and cook at 360 degrees F for 15 minutes. Divide into bowls and serve for breakfast.

Nutrition: calories 201, fat 13, fiber 2, carbs 4, protein 7

Okra and Eggs
Prep time: 5 *minutes* | *Cooking time:* 20 *minutes* | *Servings:* 4

Ingredients:
- 2 cups okra
- 1 tablespoon butter, melted
- 4 eggs, whisked
- A pinch of salt and black pepper

Directions:
Grease a pan that fits the air fryer with the butter. In a bowl, combine the okra with eggs, salt and pepper, whisk and pour into the pan. Introduce the pan in the air fryer and cook at 350 degrees F for 20 minutes. Divide the mix between plates and serve.

Nutrition: calories 220, fat 12, fiber 4, carbs 5, protein 8

Coconut Cauliflower Pudding
Prep time: 5 *minutes* | *Cooking time:* 20 *minutes* | *Servings:* 4

Ingredients:
- 1 cup cauliflower rice
- ½ cup coconut, shredded
- 3 cups coconut milk
- 2 tablespoons stevia

Directions:
In a pan that fits the air fryer, combine all the ingredients and whisk well. Introduce the in your air fryer and cook at 360 degrees F for 20 minutes. Divide into bowls and serve for breakfast.

Nutrition: calories 211, fat 11, fiber 3, carbs 4, protein 8

Celery and Bell Peppers Mix
Prep time: 5 minutes | Cooking time: 15 minutes | Servings: 4

Ingredients:
- 1 red bell pepper, roughly chopped
- 1 celery stalk, chopped
- 2 green onions, sliced
- 2 tablespoons butter, melted
- ½ cup mozzarella cheese, shredded
- A pinch of salt and black pepper
- 6 eggs, whisked

Directions:
In a bowl, mix all the ingredients except the butter and whisk well. Preheat the air fryer at 360 degrees F, add the butter, heat it up, add the celery and bell peppers mix, and cook for 15 minutes, shaking the fryer once. Divide the mix between plates and serve for breakfast.

Nutrition: calories 222, fat 12, fiber 4, carbs 5, protein 7

Tarragon and Parmesan Scramble
Prep time: 5 minutes | Cooking time: 20 minutes | Servings: 4

Ingredients:
- 8 eggs, whisked
- 2 tablespoons tarragon, chopped
- Salt and black pepper to the taste
- 2 tablespoons parmesan, grated
- ¼ cup coconut cream

Directions:
In a bowl, mix the eggs with all the ingredients and whisk. Pour this into a pan that fits your air fryer, introduce it in the preheated fryer and cook at 350 degrees F for 20 minutes, stirring often. Divide the scramble between plates and serve for breakfast.

Nutrition: calories 221, fat 12, fiber 4, carbs 5, protein 9

Watercress and Zucchini Salad
Prep time: 4 minutes | Cooking time: 15 minutes | Servings: 2

Ingredients:
- 1 cup watercress, torn
- 1 tablespoon olive oil
- 2 cups zucchini, roughly cubed
- 1 cup parmesan cheese, grated
- Cooking spray

Directions:
Grease a pan that fits the air fryer with the cooking spray, add all the ingredients except the cheese, sprinkle the cheese on top and cook at 390 degrees F for 15 minutes. Divide into bowls and serve for breakfast.

Nutrition: calories 202, fat 11, fiber 3, carbs 5, protein 4

Mustard Greens Salad
Prep time: 5 minutes | Cooking time: 15 minutes | Servings: 4

Ingredients:
- 1 teaspoon olive oil
- 2 cups mustard greens
- A pinch of salt and black pepper
- ½ pound cherry tomatoes, cubed
- 2 tablespoons chives, chopped

Directions:
Heat up your air fryer with the oil at 360 degrees F, add all the ingredients, toss, cook for 15 minutes shaking halfway, divide into bowls and serve for breakfast.

Nutrition: calories 224, fat 8, fiber 2, carbs 3, protein 7

Radish and Green Beans Salad
Prep time: 5 minutes | Cooking time: 15 minutes | Servings: 4

Ingredients:

- 1 and ¾ cups radishes, chopped
- ½ pound green beans, trimmed
- A pinch of salt and black pepper
- 4 eggs, whisked
- Cooking spray
- 1 tablespoon cilantro, chopped

Directions:

Grease a pan that fits the air fryer with the cooking spray, add all the ingredients, toss and cook at 360 degrees F for 15 minutes. Divide between plates and serve for breakfast.

Nutrition: calories 212, fat 12, fiber 3, carbs 4, protein 9

Cauliflower Rice Bowls
Prep time: 5 minutes | Cooking time: 15 minutes | Servings: 4

Ingredients:

- 12 ounces cauliflower rice
- 3 tablespoons stevia
- 2 tablespoons olive oil
- 2 tablespoons lime juice
- 1 pound fresh spinach, torn
- 1 red bell pepper, chopped

Directions:

In your air fryer, mix all the ingredients, toss, cook at 370 degrees F for 15 minutes, shaking halfway, divide between plates and serve for breakfast.

Nutrition: calories 219, fat 14, fiber 3, carbs 5, protein 7

Red Cabbage Bowls
Prep time: 5 minutes | Cooking time: 15 minutes | Servings: 4

Ingredients:
- 2 cups red cabbage, shredded
- A drizzle of olive oil
- 1 red bell pepper, sliced
- 1 small avocado, peeled, pitted and sliced
- Salt and black pepper to the taste

Directions:

Grease your air fryer with the oil, add all the ingredients, toss, cover and cook at 400 degrees F for 15 minutes. Divide into bowls and serve cold for breakfast.

Nutrition: calories 209, fat 8, fiber 2, carbs 4, protein 9

Mixed Veggie Bake
Prep time: 5 minutes | Cooking time: 20 minutes | Servings: 4

Ingredients:
- 2 garlic cloves, minced
- 1 teaspoon olive oil
- 2 celery stalks, chopped
- ½ cup white mushrooms, chopped
- ½ cup red bell pepper, chopped
- Salt and black pepper to the taste
- 1 teaspoon oregano, dried
- 7 ounces mozzarella, shredded
- 1 tablespoon lemon juice

Directions:

Preheat the Air Fryer at 350 degrees F, add the oil and heat it up. Add garlic, celery, mushrooms, bell pepper, salt, pepper, oregano, mozzarella and the lemon juice, toss and cook for 20 minutes. Divide between plates and serve for breakfast.

Nutrition: calories 230, fat 11, fiber 2, carbs 4, protein 6

Cinnamon Pudding
Prep time: 4 minutes | Cooking time: 12 minutes | Servings: 2

Ingredients:
- ½ teaspoon cinnamon powder
- ¼ teaspoon allspice, ground
- 4 tablespoons erythritol
- 4 eggs, whisked
- 2 tablespoons heavy cream
- Cooking spray

Directions:
In a bowl, mix all the ingredients except the cooking spray, whisk well and pour into a ramekin greased with cooking spray. Add the basket to your Air Fryer, put the ramekin inside and cook at 400 degrees F for 12 minutes. Divide into bowls and serve for breakfast.

Nutrition: calories 201, fat 11, fiber 2, carbs 4, protein 6

Paprika Broccoli and Eggs
Prep time: 5 minutes | Cooking time: 20 minutes | Servings: 4

Ingredients:
- 1 broccoli head, florets separated and roughly chopped
- Cooking spray
- 2 eggs, whisked
- Salt and black pepper to the taste
- 1 tablespoon sweet paprika
- 4 ounces sour cream

Directions:
Grease a pan that fits your air fryer with the cooking spray and mix all the ingredients inside. Put the pan in the Air Fryer and cook at 360 degrees F for 20 minutes. Divide between plates and serve.

Nutrition: calories 220, fat 14, fiber 2, carbs 3, protein 2

Zucchini Fritters
Prep time: 5 minutes | Cooking time: 8 minutes | Servings: 4

Ingredients:
- 8 ounces zucchinis, chopped
- 2 spring onions, chopped
- 2 eggs, whisked
- Salt and black pepper to the taste
- ¼ teaspoon sweet paprika, chopped
- Cooking spray

Directions:
In a bowl, mix all the ingredients except the cooking spray, stir well and shape medium fritters out of this mix. Put the basket in the Air Fryer, add the fritters inside, grease them with cooking spray and cook at 400 degrees F for 8 minutes. Divide the fritters between plates and serve for breakfast.

Nutrition: calories 202, fat 10, fiber 2, carbs 4, protein 5

Artichokes Omelet
Prep time: 5 minutes | Cooking time: 12 minutes | Servings: 4

Ingredients:
- 12 ounces canned artichoke hearts, drained and chopped
- Salt and black pepper to the taste
- 4 eggs, whisked
- 1 green onion, chopped
- 2 tablespoons parsley, chopped
- Cooking spray

Directions:
Grease a pan that fits your air fryer with cooking spray. In a bowl, mix all the other ingredients, whisk well and pour evenly into the pan. Introduce the pan in the air fryer, cook at 390 degrees F for 12 minutes, divide between plates and serve for breakfast.

Nutrition: calories 185, fat 8, fiber 2, carbs 5, protein 8

Fennel Frittata

Prep time: 5 minutes | Cooking time: 15 minutes | Servings: 6

Ingredients:

- 1 fennel bulb, shredded
- 6 eggs, whisked
- A pinch of salt and black pepper
- 1 teaspoon sweet paprika
- 2 teaspoons cilantro, chopped
- Cooking spray

Directions:

In a bowl, mix all the ingredients except the cooking spray and stir well. Grease a baking pan with the cooking spray, pour the frittata mix and spread well. Put the pan in the Air Fryer and cook at 370 degrees F for 15 minutes. Divide between plates and serve them for breakfast.

Nutrition: calories 200, fat 12, fiber 1, carbs 5, protein 8

Eggs and Spinach Salad

Prep time: 5 minutes | Cooking time: 10 minutes | Servings: 4

Ingredients:

- 1 tablespoon lime juice
- 4 eggs, hard boiled, peeled and sliced
- 2 cups baby spinach
- Salt and black pepper to the taste
- 3 tablespoons heavy cream
- 2 tablespoons olive oil

Directions:

In your Air Fryer, mix the spinach with cream, eggs, salt and pepper, cover and cook at 360 degrees F for 6 minutes. Transfer this to a bowl, add the lime juice and oil, toss and serve for breakfast.

Nutrition: calories 200, fat 7, fiber 3, carbs 4, protein 7

Bok Choy and Spinach Mix
Prep time: 5 minutes | Cooking time: 15 minutes | Servings: 4

Ingredients:
- 7 ounces bok choy, torn
- 7 ounces baby spinach, torn
- 2 tablespoons olive oil
- 2 eggs, whisked
- 2 tablespoons coconut cream
- 3 ounces mozzarella, shredded
- Salt and black pepper to the taste

Directions:
In your Air Fryer, combine all the ingredients except the mozzarella and toss them gently. Sprinkle the mozzarella on top, cook at 360 degrees F for 15 minutes, divide between plates and serve.
Nutrition: calories 200, fat 12, fiber 2, carbs 3, protein 8

Artichokes and Zucchini Mix
Prep time: 5 minutes | Cooking time: 20 minutes | Servings: 4

Ingredients:
- 8 ounces canned artichokes, drained and chopped
- 2 zucchinis, sliced
- 4 spring onions, chopped
- 2 tomatoes, cut into quarters
- 4 eggs, whisked
- Cooking spray
- Salt and black pepper to the taste

Directions:
Grease a pan with cooking spray, and mix all the other ingredients inside. Put the pan in the Air Fryer and cook at 350 degrees F for 20 minutes. Divide between plates and serve.
Nutrition: calories 210, fat 11, fiber 3, carbs 4, protein 6

Cheesy Tomatoes Mix

Prep time: 5 minutes | Cooking time: 15 minutes | Servings: 4

Ingredients:

- 1 pound cherry tomatoes, halved
- 1 cup mozzarella, shredded
- Cooking spray
- Salt and black pepper to the taste
- 1 teaspoon basil, chopped

Directions:

Grease the tomatoes with the cooking spray, season with salt and pepper, sprinkle the mozzarella on top, place them all in your air fryer's basket, cook at 330 degrees F for 15 minutes, divide into bowls, sprinkle the basil on top and serve.

Nutrition: calories 140, fat 7, fiber 3, carbs 4, protein 5

Blackberries Bowls

Prep time: 5 minutes | Cooking time: 15 minutes | Servings: 4

Ingredients:

- 1 and ½ cups coconut milk
- ½ cup blackberries
- 2 teaspoon stevia
- ½ cup coconut, shredded

Directions:

In your air fryer's pan, mix all the ingredients, stir, cover and cook at 360 degrees F for 15 minutes. Divide into bowls and serve for breakfast.

Nutrition: calories 171, fat 4, fiber 2, carbs 3, protein 5

Raspberries Oatmeal

Prep time: 5 minutes | Cooking time: 15 minutes | Servings: 4

Ingredients:

- 2 cups almond milk
- ½ cups raspberries
- 1 and ½ cups coconut, shredded
- ½ teaspoon cinnamon powder
- ¼ teaspoon nutmeg, ground
- 2 teaspoons stevia
- Cooking spray

Directions:

Grease the air fryer's pan with cooking spray, mix all the ingredients inside, cover and cook at 360 degrees F for 15 minutes. Divide into bowls and serve for breakfast.

Nutrition: calories 172, fat 5, fiber 2, carbs 4, protein 6

Strawberries Oatmeal
Prep time: 5 minutes | Cooking time: 15 minutes | Ingredients: 4

Ingredients:

- 2 cups coconut milk
- ¼ cup strawberries
- ¼ teaspoon vanilla extract
- ½ cup coconut, shredded
- 2 teaspoons stevia
- Cooking spray

Directions:

Grease the Air Fryer's pan with the cooking spray, add all the ingredients inside and toss. Cook at 365 degrees F for 15 minutes, divide into bowls and serve for breakfast.

Nutrition: calories 142, fat 7, fiber 2, carbs 3, protein 5

Olives and Tomatoes Eggs
Prep time: 5 minutes | Cooking time: 15 minutes | Servings: 4

Ingredients:

- 1 cup kalamata olives, pitted
- 1 cup cherry tomatoes, cubed
- 4 eggs, whisked
- A pinch of salt
- Cooking spray

Directions:

Grease the air fryer with cooking spray, add all the ingredients, toss, cover and cook at 365 degrees F for 10 minutes. Divide between plates and serve for breakfast.

Nutrition: calories 182, fat 6, fiber 2, carbs 4, protein 8

Green Beans and Olives Mix
Prep time: 5 minutes | Cooking time: 20 minutes | Servings: 2

Ingredients:

- 1 cup green beans, halved
- 2 spring onions, chopped
- 4 eggs, whisked
- Salt and black pepper
- ¼ teaspoon cumin, ground

Directions:

Preheat the air fryer at 360 degrees F, add all the ingredients, toss, cover, cook for 20 minutes, divide between plates and serve for breakfast.

Nutrition: calories 183, fat 8, fiber 2, carbs 3, protein 7

Lemony Raspberries Bowls

Prep time: 5 minutes | Cooking time: 12 minutes | Servings: 2

Ingredients:

- 1 cup raspberries
- 2 tablespoons lemon juice
- 2 tablespoons butter
- 1 teaspoon cinnamon powder

Directions:

In your air fryer, mix all the ingredients, toss, cover, cook at 350 degrees F for 12 minutes, divide into bowls and serve for breakfast.

Nutrition: calories 208, fat 6, fiber 9, carbs 14, protein 3

Ketogenic Air Fryer Lunch Recipes

Tomato and Avocado Mix
Prep time: 3 minutes | Cooking time: 5 minutes | Servings: 4

Ingredients:

- 1./3 cup coconut cream
- ½ pound cherry tomatoes, halved
- 2 avocados, pitted, peeled and cubed
- 1 and ¼ cup lettuce, torn
- A pinch of salt and black pepper
- Cooking spray

Directions:

Grease the air fryer with cooking spray, combine the tomatoes with avocados, salt, pepper and the cream and cook at 350 degrees F for 5 minutes shaking once. In a salad bowl, mix the lettuce with the tomatoes and avocado mix, toss and serve for lunch.

Nutrition: calories 226, fat 12, fiber 2, carbs 4, protein 8

Pork Pan
Prep time: 5 minutes | Cooking time: 20 minutes | Servings: 4

Ingredients:

- 1 pound pork stew meat, ground
- 1 cup mushrooms, sliced
- 2 spring onions, chopped
- Salt and black pepper to the taste
- 1 teaspoon Italian seasoning
- ½ teaspoon garlic powder
- 1 tablespoon olive oil

Directions:

Heat up a pan that fits the air fryer with the oil over medium high heat, add the meat and brown for 3-4 minutes. Add the rest of the ingredients, stir, put the pan in the Air Fryer, cover and cook at 360 degrees F for 15 minutes. Divide between plates and serve for lunch.

Nutrition: calories 220, fat 12, fiber 2, carbs 4, protein 7

Spring Onions and Chicken Breast
Prep time: 5 minutes | Cooking time: 30 minutes | Servings: 4

Ingredients:

- 1 teaspoon olive oil
- 4 spring onions, chopped
- 2 chicken breasts, skinless, boneless and cubed
- Salt and black pepper to the taste
- 1 and ½ cups parmesan cheese, grated
- ½ cup tomato puree

Directions:

Preheat your air fryer at 400 degrees F, add half of the oil and the spring onions and fry them for 8 minutes, shaking the fryer halfway. Add the rest of the ingredients, toss, cook at 370 degrees F for 22 minutes, shaking the fryer halfway as well. Divide between plates and serve for lunch.

Nutrition: calories 270, fat 14, fiber 2, carbs 6, protein 12

Pork Bowls
Prep time: 10 minutes | Cooking time: 15 minutes | Servings: 4

Ingredients:

- 2 eggs, whisked
- 1 and ½ pounds pork meat, ground
- 2 teaspoons olive oil
- ½ cup tomato puree
- Salt and black pepper to the taste

Directions:

Heat up a pan that fits the Air Fryer with the oil over medium-high heat, add the meat and brown for 3-4 minutes. Add the rest of the ingredients, toss, put the pan in the machine and cook at 370 degrees F for 12 minutes. Divide into bowls and serve for lunch with a side salad.

Nutrition: calories 270, fat 13, fiber 2, carbs 6, protein 8

Lemony Chicken Thighs

Prep time: 10 minutes | Cooking time: 35 minutes | Servings: 6

Ingredients:

- 3 pounds chicken thighs, bone-in
- ½ cup butter, melted
- 1 tablespoon smoked paprika
- 1 teaspoon lemon juice

Directions:

In a bowl, mix the chicken thighs with the paprika, toss, put all the pieces in your air fryer's basket and cook them at 360 degrees F for 25 minutes shaking the fryer from time to time and basting the meat with the butter. Divide between plates and serve.

Nutrition: calories 261, fat 16, fiber 3, carbs 5, protein 12

Mustard Chicken Thighs

Prep time: 5 minutes | Cooking time: 30 minutes | Servings: 4

Ingredients:

- 1 and ½ pounds chicken thighs, bone-in
- 2 tablespoons Dijon mustard
- A pinch of salt and black pepper
- Cooking spray

Directions:

In a bowl, mix the chicken thighs with all the other ingredients and toss. Put the chicken in your Air Fryer's basket and cook at 370 degrees F for 30 minutes shaking halfway. Serve these chicken thighs for lunch.

Nutrition: calories 253, fat 17, fiber 3, carbs 6, protein 12

Hot Eggplant Bake
Prep time: 5 minutes | Cooking time: 20 minutes | Servings: 4

Ingredients:
- 2 eggplants, cubed
- 1 hot chili pepper, chopped
- 4 spring onions, chopped
- ½ pound cherry tomatoes, cubed
- Salt and black pepper to the taste
- 2 teaspoons olive oil
- ½ cup cilantro, chopped
- 4 garlic cloves, minced

Directions:
Grease a baking pan that fits the air fryer with the oil, and mix all the ingredients in the pan. Put the pan in the preheated air fryer and cook at 380 degrees F for 20 minutes, divide into bowls and serve for lunch.

Nutrition: calories 232, fat 12, fiber 3, carbs 5, protein 10

Beef and Tomato Sauce
Prep time: 5 minutes | Cooking time: 20 minutes | Servings: 4

Ingredients:
- 1 pound lean beef meat, cubed and browned
- 2 garlic cloves, minced
- Salt and black pepper to the taste
- Cooking spray
- 16 ounces tomato sauce

Directions:
Preheat the Air Fryer at 400 degrees F, add the pan inside, grease it with cooking spray, add the meat and all the other ingredients, toss and cook for 20 minutes. Divide into bowls and serve for lunch.

Nutrition: calories 270, fat 15, fiber 3, carbs 6, protein 12

Oregano Beef Mix
Prep time: 5 minutes | Cooking time: 20 minutes | Servings: 4

Ingredients:

- 14 ounces beef, cubed
- 7 ounces tomato sauce
- 1 tablespoon chives, chopped
- 2 tablespoons parmesan cheese, grated
- 1 tablespoon oregano, chopped
- 1 tablespoon olive oil
- Salt and black pepper to the taste

Directions:

Grease a pan that fits the air fryer with the oil and mix all the ingredients except the parmesan. Sprinkle the parmesan on top, put the pan in the machine and cook at 380 degrees F for 20 minutes. Divide between plates and serve for lunch.

Nutrition: calories 280, fat 14, fiber 4, carbs 6, protein 15

Salmon and Kale Salad
Prep time: 5 minutes | Cooking time: 8 minutes | Servings: 4

Ingredients:

- 4 salmon fillets, boneless
- 2 tablespoons olive oil
- Salt and black pepper to the taste
- 3 cups kale leaves, shredded
- 2 teaspoons balsamic vinegar

Directions:

Put the fish in your air fryer's basket, season with salt and pepper, drizzle half of the oil over them, cook at 400 degrees F for 4 minutes on each side, cool down and cut into medium cubes. In a bowl, mix the kale with salt, pepper, vinegar, the rest of the oil and the salmon, toss gently and serve for lunch.

Nutrition: calories 240, fat 14, fiber 3, carbs 5, protein 10

Turkey and Bok Choy
Prep time: 5 minutes | *Cooking time:* 20 minutes | *Servings:* 4

Ingredients:
- 1 turkey breast, boneless, skinless and cubed
- 2 teaspoons olive oil
- ½ teaspoon sweet paprika
- Salt and black pepper to the taste
- 2 cups bok choy, torn and steamed
- 1 tablespoon balsamic vinegar

Directions:
In a bowl, mix the turkey with the oil, paprika, salt and pepper, toss, transfer them to your Air Fryer's basket and cook at 350 degrees F for 20 minutes. In a salad, mix the turkey with all the other ingredients, toss and serve for lunch.

Nutrition: calories 250, fat 13, fiber 3, carbs 6, protein 14

Paprika Cod Mix
Prep time: 5 minutes | *Cooking time:* 12 minutes | *Servings:* 4

Ingredients:
- 2 tablespoons fresh cilantro, minced
- 1 pound cod fillets, boneless, skinless and cubed
- 1 spring onion, chopped
- Salt and black pepper to the taste
- ½ teaspoon sweet paprika
- ½ teaspoon oregano, ground
- A drizzle of olive oil
- 2 cups baby arugula

Directions:
In a bowl, mix the cod with salt, pepper, paprika, oregano and the oil, toss, transfer the cubes to your air fryer's basket and cook at 360 degrees F for 12 minutes. In a salad bowl, mix the cod with the remaining ingredients, toss, divide between plates and serve.

Nutrition: calories 240, fat 11, fiber 3, carbs 5, protein 8

Pork Stew
Prep time: 5 minutes | Cooking time: 30 minutes | Servings: 4

Ingredients:
- 2 pounds pork stew meat, cubed
- 2 zucchinis, cubed
- 1 eggplant, cubed
- Salt and black pepper to the taste
- ½ cup beef stock
- ½ teaspoon smoked paprika
- A handful cilantro, chopped

Directions:
In a pan that fits your air fryer, mix all the ingredients, toss, introduce in your air fryer and cook at 370 degrees F for 30 minutes. Divide into bowls and serve right away.

Nutrition: calories 245, fat 12, fiber 2, carbs 5, protein 14

Chili Salmon and Shrimp Bowls
Prep time: 5 minutes | Cooking time: 12 minutes | Servings: 4

Ingredients:
- 2 salmon fillets, boneless, skinless and cubed
- 8 ounces shrimp, peeled and deveined
- Salt and black pepper to the taste
- 5 garlic cloves, minced
- 1 teaspoon sweet paprika
- 2 tablespoons olive oil

Directions:
In a pan that fits the air fryer, combine all the ingredients, toss, cover and cook at 370 degrees F for 12 minutes. Divide into bowls and serve for lunch.

Nutrition: calories 270, fat 8, fiber 2, carbs 4, protein 7

Cheese Eggplant Bowls
Prep time: 5 minutes | Cooking time: 15 minutes | Servings: 4

Ingredients:
- 2 cups eggplants, cubed
- 1 cup tomato puree
- 1 teaspoon olive oil
- 1 cup mozzarella, shredded

Directions:
In a pan that fits the air fryer, combine all the ingredients except the mozzarella and toss. Sprinkle the cheese on top, introduce the pan in the machine and cook at 390 degrees F for 15 minutes. Divide between plates and serve for lunch.

Nutrition: calories 220, fat 9, fiber 2, carbs 6, protein 9

Cilantro Chicken and Asparagus
Prep time: 5 minutes | Cooking time: 20 minutes | Servings: 4

Ingredients:
- 4 chicken breasts, skinless, boneless and halved
- 1 tablespoon sweet paprika
- 1 bunch asparagus, trimmed and halved
- 1 tablespoon olive oil
- Salt and black pepper to the taste

Directions:
In a bowl, mix all the ingredients, toss, put them in your Air Fryer's basket and cook at 390 degrees F for 20 minutes. Divide between plates and serve for lunch.

Nutrition: calories 230, fat 11, fiber 3, carbs 5, protein 12

Turkey and Zucchini Casserole
Prep time: 5 minutes | *Cooking time:* 25 minutes | *Servings:* 4

Ingredients:

- 2 tablespoons butter, melted
- 12 ounces cream cheese, soft
- 2 cups turkey breasts, skinless, boneless and cut into strips
- 1 cups zucchinis, sliced
- 2 teaspoons sweet paprika
- 6 ounces cheddar cheese, grated
- ¼ cup cilantro, chopped
- Salt and black pepper to the taste

Directions:

In a baking dish that fits your air fryer, mix the butter with turkey, cream cheese and all the other ingredients except the cheddar cheese. Sprinkle the cheddar on top, put the dish in your air fryer and cook at 360 degrees F for 25 minutes. Divide between plates and serve for lunch.

Nutrition: calories 280, fat 10, fiber 2, carbs 4, protein 12

Creamy Chicken
Prep time: 4 minutes | *Cooking time:* 20 minutes | *Servings:* 4

Ingredients:

- 4 chicken breasts, skinless, boneless and cubed
- Salt and black pepper to the taste
- ¼ cup coconut cream
- 1 teaspoon olive oil
- 1 and ½ teaspoon sweet paprika

Directions:

Grease a pan that fits your air fryer with the oil, mix all the ingredients inside, introduce the pan in the fryer and cook at 370 degrees F for 17 minutes. Divide between plates and serve for lunch.

Nutrition: calories 250, fat 12, fiber 2, carbs 5, protein 11

Pork and Mustard Greens Bowls
Prep time: 5 minutes | Cooking time: 20 minutes | Servings: 4

Ingredients:
- ½ pound pork stew meat, cubed
- ¼ cup tomato puree
- 1 tablespoon olive oil
- 2 cups mustard greens
- 1 yellow bell pepper, chopped
- 2 green onions, chopped
- Salt and black pepper to the taste

Directions:
In a pan that fits your air fryer, mix all the ingredients, toss, introduce the pan in the air fryer and cook at 370 degrees F for 20 minutes. Divide into bowls and serve for lunch.

Nutrition: calories 265, fat 12, fiber 3, carbs 5, protein 14

Celery and Chicken Stew
Prep time: 5 minutes | Cooking time: 30 minutes | Servings: 6

Ingredients:
- 1 tablespoon butter, soft
- 4 celery stalks, chopped
- 2 red bell peppers, chopped
- 1 pound chicken breasts, skinless, boneless and cubed
- 2 teaspoons garlic, minced
- Salt and black pepper to the taste
- ½ cup coconut cream

Directions:
Grease a baking dish that fits your air fryer with the butter, add all the ingredients in the pan and toss them. Introduce the dish in the fryer, cook at 360 degrees F for 30 minutes, divide into bowls and serve for lunch.

Nutrition: calories 246, fat 12, fiber 2, carbs 6, protein 12

Zucchini Stew
Prep time: 5 *minutes* | *Cooking time:* 12 *minutes* | *Servings:* 4

Ingredients:
- ¼ cup tomato sauce
- 1 tablespoon olive oil
- 8 zucchinis, roughly cubed
- Salt and black pepper to the taste
- ¼ teaspoon rosemary, dried
- ½ teaspoon basil, chopped

Directions:
Grease a pan that fits your air fryer with the oil, add all the ingredients, toss, introduce the pan in the fryer and cook at 350 degrees F for 12 minutes. Divide into bowls and serve for lunch.

Nutrition: calories 200, fat 6, fiber 2, carbs 4, protein 6

Turkey and Mushroom Stew
Prep time: 5 *minutes* | *Cooking time:* 25 *minutes* | *Servings:* 4

Ingredients:
- ½ pound brown mushrooms, sliced
- Salt and black pepper to the taste
- ¼ cup tomato sauce
- 1 turkey breast, skinless, boneless, cubed and browned
- 1 tablespoon parsley, chopped

Directions:
In a pan that fits your air fryer, mix the turkey with the mushrooms, salt, pepper and tomato sauce, toss, introduce in the fryer and cook at 350 degrees F for 25 minutes. Divide into bowls and serve for lunch with parsley sprinkled on top.

Nutrition: calories 220, fat 12, fiber 2, carbs 5, protein 12

Chili Pork Stew
Prep time: 5 minutes | *Cooking time:* 25 minutes | *Servings:* 4

Ingredients:
- 1 and ½ pound pork stew meat, cubed
- ½ cup cilantro, chopped
- ½ cup green onions, chopped
- ½ cup tomato sauce
- A drizzle of olive oil
- 2 teaspoons chili powder

Directions:
Heat up a pan that fits the air fryer with the oil over medium-high heat, add the meat and brown for 5 minutes. Add the rest of the ingredients, toss, introduce the pan in the air fryer and cook at 370 degrees F for 20 minutes. Divide into and serve for lunch

Nutrition: calories 285, fat 14, fiber 4, carbs 6, protein 15

Buttery Cod Bake
Prep time: 5 minutes | *Cooking time:* 12 minutes | *Servings:* 4

Ingredients:
- 3 tablespoons butter, melted
- 2 tablespoons parsley, chopped
- ¼ cup tomato sauce
- 8 cherry tomatoes, halved
- 2 cod fillets, boneless, skinless and cubed
- Salt and black pepper to the taste

Directions:
In a baking pan that fits the air fryer, combine all the ingredients, toss, put the pan in the machine and cook the mix at 390 degrees F for 12 minutes. Divide the mix into bowls and serve for lunch.

Nutrition: calories 232, fat 8, fiber 2, carbs 5, protein 11

Turkey and Broccoli Stew
Prep time: 5 minutes | Cooking time: 25 minutes | Servings: 4

Ingredients:

- 1 turkey breast, skinless, boneless and cubed
- 1 tablespoon olive oil
- 1 broccoli head, florets separated
- 1 cup tomato sauce
- Salt and black pepper to the taste
- 1 tablespoon parsley, chopped

Directions:

In a baking dish that fits your air fryer, mix the turkey with the rest of the ingredients except the parsley, toss, introduce the dish in the fryer, bake at 380 degrees F for 25 minutes, divide into bowls, sprinkle the parsley on top and serve.

Nutrition: calories 250, fat 11, fiber 2, carbs 6, protein 12

Garlicky Pork Stew
Prep time: 5 minutes | Cooking time: 25 minutes | Servings: 4

Ingredients:

- 1 pound pork stew meat, cubed
- 3 garlic cloves, minced
- ¼ cup tomato sauce
- 1 cup spinach, torn
- ½ teaspoon olive oil

Directions:

In pan that fits your air fryer, mix the pork with the other ingredients except the spinach, toss, introduce in the fryer and cook at 370 degrees F for 15 minutes. Add the spinach, toss, cook for 10 minutes more, divide into bowls and serve for lunch.

Nutrition: calories 290, fat 14, fiber 3, carbs 5, protein 13

Shrimp Stew
Prep time: 5 minutes | Cooking time: 12 minutes | Servings: 4

Ingredients:
- 1 red bell pepper, chopped
- 14 ounces chicken stock
- 2 tablespoons tomato sauce
- 3 spring onions, chopped
- 1 and ½ pounds shrimp, peeled and deveined
- Salt and black pepper to the taste
- 1 tablespoon olive oil

Directions:
In your air fryer's pan greased with the oil, mix the shrimp and the other ingredients, toss, introduce the pan in the machine, and cook at 360 degrees F for 12 minutes, stirring halfway. Divide into bowls and serve for lunch.

Nutrition: calories 223, fat 12, fiber 2, carbs 5, protein 9

Beef and Pork Bake
Prep time: 5 minutes | Cooking time: 30 minutes | Servings: 4

Ingredients:
- 1 pound lean beef, cubed
- 1 pound pork stew meat, cubed
- 1 tablespoon spring onions, chopped
- 2 tablespoons tomato sauce
- A drizzle of olive oil
- A pinch of salt and black pepper
- ¼ teaspoon sweet paprika

Directions:
Heat up a pan that fits the air fryer with the oil over medium-high heat, add the pork and beef meat and brown for 5 minutes. Add the remaining ingredients, toss, introduce the pan in the air fryer and cook at 390 degrees F for 25 minutes. Divide the mix between plates and serve for lunch with a side salad.

Nutrition: calories 275, fat 14, fiber 2, carbs 6, protein 14

Rosemary Lamb and Spinach
Prep time: 5 minutes | Cooking time: 30 minutes | Servings: 4

Ingredients:
- 1 tablespoon olive oil
- 2 garlic clove, minced
- 1 tablespoon rosemary, chopped
- ¼ cup tomato sauce
- 1 cup baby spinach
- 1 and ½ pounds lamb, cubed
- Salt and black pepper to the taste

Directions:
Heat up a pan that fits the air fryer with the oil over medium heat, add the lamb and garlic and brown for 5 minutes. Add the rest of the ingredients except the spinach, introduce the pan in the fryer and cook at 390 degrees F for 15 minutes, shaking the machine halfway. Add the spinach, cook for 10 minutes more, divide between plates and serve for lunch.

Nutrition: calories 257, fat 12, fiber 3, carbs 6, protein 14

Pork and Okra Stew
Prep time: 5 minutes | Cooking time: 20 minutes | Servings: 4

Ingredients:
- 1 and ½ pounds pork stew meat, cubed and browned
- 2 teaspoons sweet paprika
- 1 tablespoon olive oil
- 1 cup okra
- Salt and black pepper to the taste
- 3 garlic cloves, minced

Directions:
In your air fryer's pan, combine the meat with the remaining ingredients, toss, cover and cook at 370 degrees F for 20 minutes. Divide the stew into bowls and serve.

Nutrition: calories 275, fat 12, fiber 4, carbs 6, protein 15

Lamb and Eggplant Stew
Prep time: 5 minutes | Cooking time: 30 minutes | Servings: 4

Ingredients:
- 1 cup eggplant, cubed
- 2 garlic cloves, minced
- 3 celery ribs, chopped
- ½ cups tomato sauce
- 1 pound lamb stew meat, cubed
- 1 tablespoon olive oil
- Salt and black pepper to the taste

Directions:
Heat up a pan that fits the air fryer with the oil over medium-high heat, add the lamb, salt, pepper and the garlic and brown for 5 minutes. Add the rest of the ingredients, toss, introduce the pan in the machine and cook at 370 degrees F for 25 minutes. Divide into bowls and serve for lunch.

Nutrition: calories 235, fat 14, fiber 3, carbs 5, protein 14

Okra and Zucchini Stew
Prep time: 5 minutes | Cooking time: 20 minutes | Servings: 4

Ingredients:
- 1 cup okra
- 4 zucchinis, roughly cubed
- 1 teaspoon oregano, dried
- 2 green bell peppers, cut into strips
- 2 garlic cloves, minced
- Salt and black pepper to the taste
- 7 ounces tomato sauce
- 2 tablespoons olive oil
- 2 tablespoons cilantro, chopped

Directions:
In a pan that fits your air fryer, combine all the ingredients for the stew, toss, introduce the pan in the air fryer, cook the stew at 350 degrees F for 20 minutes, divide into bowls, and serve.

Nutrition: calories 230, fat 5, fiber 2, carbs 4, protein 8

Thyme Eggplant and Green Beans
Prep time: 5 minutes | Cooking time: 20 minutes | Servings: 6

Ingredients:

- 1 pound green beans, trimmed and halved
- 2 eggplants, cubed
- 1 cup veggie stock
- 1 tablespoon olive oil
- 1 red chili pepper
- 1 red bell pepper, chopped
- ½ teaspoon thyme, dried
- Salt and black pepper to the taste

Directions:

In a pan that fits your air fryer, mix all the ingredients, toss, introduce the pan in the machine and cook at 350 degrees F for 20 minutes. Divide into bowls and serve for lunch.

Nutrition: calories 180, fat 3, fiber 2, carbs 5, protein 7

Bell Peppers Stew
Prep time: 5 minutes | Cooking time: 15 minutes | Servings: 4

Ingredients:

- 2 red bell peppers, cut into wedges
- 2 green bell peppers, cut into wedges
- 2 yellow bell peppers, cut into wedges
- ½ cup tomato sauce
- 1 tablespoon chili powder
- 2 teaspoons cumin, ground
- ¼ teaspoon sweet paprika
- Salt and black pepper to the taste

Directions:

In a pan that fits your air fryer, mix all the ingredients, toss, introduce the pan in the machine and cook at 370 degrees F for 15 minutes. Divide into bowls and serve for lunch.

Nutrition: calories 190, fat 4, fiber 2, carbs 4, protein 7

Summer Okra and Green Beans Stew
Prep time: 5 minutes | Cooking time: 15 minutes | Servings: 4

Ingredients:
- 1 pound green beans, halved
- 1 cup okra
- 1 tablespoon thyme, chopped
- 3 tablespoons tomato sauce
- Salt and black pepper to the taste
- 4 garlic cloves, minced

Directions:
In a pan that fits your air fryer, mix all the ingredients, toss, introduce the pan in the air fryer and cook at 370 degrees F for 15 minutes. Divide the stew into bowls and serve.

Nutrition: calories 183, fat 5, fiber 2, carbs 4, protein 8

Chicken and Okra Stew
Prep time: 5 minutes | Cooking time: 20 minutes | Servings: 4

Ingredients:
- 2 cups okra
- 2 garlic cloves, minced
- 1 pound chicken breasts, skinless, boneless and cubed
- 4 tomatoes, cubed
- 1 tablespoon olive oil
- 1 teaspoon rosemary, dried
- Salt and black pepper to the taste
- 1 tablespoon parsley, chopped

Directions:
Heat up a pan that fits your air fryer with the oil over medium-high heat, add the chicken, garlic, rosemary, salt and pepper, toss and brown for 5 minutes. Add the remaining ingredients, toss again, place the pan in the air fryer and cook at 380 degrees F for 15 minutes more. Divide the stew into bowls and serve for lunch.

Nutrition: calories 220, fat 13, fiber 3, carbs 5, protein 11

Spinach and Shrimp Mix

Prep time: 5 minutes | Cooking time: 15 minutes | Servings: 4

Ingredients:

- 2 cups baby spinach
- ¼ cup veggie stock
- 2 tomatoes, cubed
- 1 tablespoon garlic, minced
- 15 ounces shrimp, peeled and deveined
- 4 spring onions, chopped
- ½ teaspoon cumin, ground
- 1 tablespoon lemon juice
- 2 tablespoons cilantro, chopped
- Salt and black pepper to the taste

Directions:

In a pan that fits your air fryer, mix all the ingredients except the cilantro, toss, introduce in the air fryer and cook at 360 degrees F for 15 minutes. Add the cilantro, stir, divide into bowls and serve for lunch.

Nutrition: calories 201, fat 8, fiber 2, carbs 4, protein 8

Tomato Stew

Prep time: 5 minutes | Cooking time: 15 minutes | Servings: 4

Ingredients:

- 4 spring onions, chopped
- 25 ounces canned tomatoes, cubed
- 1 teaspoon sweet paprika
- Salt and black pepper to the taste
- 2 red bell peppers, cubed
- 1 tablespoon cilantro, chopped

Directions:

In a pan that fits your air fryer, mix all the ingredients, toss, introduce the pan in the fryer and cook at 360 degrees F for 15 minutes. Divide into bowls and serve for lunch.

Nutrition: calories 185, fat 3, fiber 2, carbs 4, protein 9

Fennel and Tomato Stew
Prep time: 5 minutes | Cooking time: 15 minutes | Servings: 4

Ingredients:
- 2 cups tomatoes, cubed
- 2 fennel bulbs, shredded
- ½ cup chicken stock
- 2 tablespoons tomato puree
- 1 red bell pepper, chopped
- 2 garlic cloves, minced
- 1 teaspoon sweet paprika
- 1 teaspoon rosemary, dried
- Salt and black pepper to the taste

Directions:
In a pan that fits your air fryer, mix all the ingredients, toss, introduce in the fryer and cook at 380 degrees F for 15 minutes. Divide the stew into bowls and serve for lunch.

Nutrition: calories 184, fat 7, fiber 2, carbs 3, protein 8

Okra Casserole
Prep time: 5 minutes | Cooking time: 20 minutes | Servings: 4

Ingredients:
- 1 teaspoon olive oil
- 3 cups okra
- 2 red bell peppers, cubed
- Salt and black pepper to the taste
- 2 tomatoes, chopped
- 3 garlic cloves, minced
- ¼ cup tomato puree
- 2 teaspoons coriander, ground
- 1 tablespoon cilantro, chopped
- ½ cup cheddar, shredded

Directions:
Grease a heat proof dish that fits your air fryer with the oil, add all the ingredients except the cilantro and the cheese and toss them really gently. Sprinkle the cheese and the cilantro on top, introduce the dish in the fryer and cook at 390 degrees F for 20 minutes. Divide between plates and serve for lunch.

Nutrition: calories 221, fat 7, fiber 2, carbs 4, protein 9

Courgettes Casserole
Prep time: 5 minutes | Cooking time: 20 minutes | Servings: 4

Ingredients:

- 1 tablespoon olive oil
- 2 spring onions, chopped
- 3 garlic cloves, minced
- 1 teaspoon smoked paprika
- 1 tablespoon thyme, dried
- 2 celery sticks, sliced
- 1 yellow bell pepper, chopped
- 14 ounces cherry tomatoes, cubed
- 2 courgettes, sliced
- ½ cup mozzarella, shredded

Directions:

In a baking dish that fits your air fryer, mix all the ingredients except the cheese and toss. Sprinkle the cheese on top, introduce the dish in your air fryer and cook at 380 degrees F for 20 minutes. Divide between plates and serve for lunch.

Nutrition: calories 254, fat 12, fiber 2, carbs 4, protein 11

Basil Chicken Bites
Prep time: 5 minutes | Cooking time: 25 minutes | Servings: 4

Ingredients:

- 1 and ½ pound chicken breasts, skinless, boneless and cubed
- Salt and black pepper to the taste
- ½ cup chicken stock
- 2 teaspoons smoked paprika
- ½ teaspoon basil, dried

Directions:

In a pan that fits the air fryer, combine all the ingredients, toss, introduce the pan in the fryer and cook at 390 degrees F for 25 minutes. Divide between plates and serve for lunch with a side salad.

Nutrition: calories 223, fat 12, fiber 2, carbs 5, protein 13

Cabbage and Tomatoes Stew
Prep time: 5 minutes | *Cooking time:* 20 minutes | *Servings:* 4

Ingredients:

- 14 ounces canned tomatoes, chopped
- 1 green cabbage head, shredded
- Salt and black pepper to the taste
- 1 tablespoon sweet paprika
- 4 ounces chicken stock
- 2 tablespoon dill, chopped

Directions:

In a pan that fits your air fryer, mix the cabbage with the tomatoes and all the other ingredients except the dill, toss, introduce the pan in the fryer, and cook at 380 degrees F for 20 minutes. Divide into bowls and serve with dill sprinkled on top.

Nutrition: calories 200, fat 8, fiber 3, carbs 4, protein 6

Broccoli Stew
Prep time: 5 minutes | *Cooking time:* 15 minutes | *Servings:* 4

Ingredients:

- 1 broccoli head, florets separated
- 3 tablespoons chicken stock
- ¾ cup tomato sauce
- 3 spring onions, chopped
- ¼ cup celery, chopped
- Salt and black pepper to the taste

Directions:

In a pan that fits your air fryer, mix all the ingredients, toss, introduce the pan in your fryer and cook at 380 degrees F for 15 minutes. Divide into bowls and serve for lunch.

Nutrition: calories 183, fat 4, fiber 2, carbs 4, protein 7

Cauliflower and Zucchini Stew
Prep time: 5 minutes | Cooking time: 20 minutes | Servings: 4

Ingredients:

- 1 and ½ cups zucchinis, sliced
- 1 tablespoon olive oil
- Salt and black pepper to the taste
- 1 tablespoon balsamic vinegar
- 1 cauliflower head, florets separated
- 2 green onions, chopped
- 1 handful parsley leaves, chopped
- ½ cup tomato puree

Directions:

In a pan that fits your air fryer, mix the zucchinis with the rest of the ingredients except the parsley, toss, introduce the pan in the air fryer and cook at 380 degrees F for 20 minutes. Divide into bowls and serve for lunch with parsley sprinkled on top.

Nutrition: calories 193, fat 5, fiber 2, carbs 4, protein 7

Olives and Spinach Mix
Prep time: 5 minutes | Cooking time: 20 minutes | Servings: 4

Ingredients:

- 2 cups black olives, pitted and halved
- 1 red bell pepper, chopped
- 3 celery stalks, chopped
- Salt and black pepper to the taste
- 4 cups spinach, torn
- 2 tomatoes, chopped
- ½ cup tomato puree

Directions:

In a pan that fits your air fryer, mix all the ingredients except the spinach, toss, introduce the pan in the air fryer and cook at 370 degrees F for 15 minutes. Add the spinach, toss, cook for 5-6 minutes more, divide into bowls and serve.

Nutrition: calories 193, fat 6, fiber 2, carbs 4, protein 6

Pork and Red Cabbage Stew
Prep time: 5 minutes | Cooking time: 30 minutes | Servings: 4

Ingredients:
- 1 and ½ pounds pork stew meat, cubed
- 1 red cabbage, shredded
- 1 tablespoon olive oil
- Salt and black pepper to the taste
- 2 chili peppers, chopped
- 4 garlic cloves, minced
- ½ cup veggie stock
- ¼ cup tomato puree

Directions:
Heat up a pan that fits the air fryer with the oil over medium heat, add the meat, chili peppers and the garlic, stir and brown for 5 minutes. Add the rest of the ingredients, toss, introduce the pan in the fryer and cook at 380 degrees F for 20 minutes. Divide the into bowls and serve for lunch.

Nutrition: calories 232, fat 11, fiber 3, carbs 5, protein 12

Leeks and Eggplant Stew
Prep time: 5 minutes | Cooking time: 20 minutes | Servings: 4

Ingredients:
- 2 big eggplants, roughly cubed
- 1 cup veggie stock
- 3 leeks, sliced
- 2 tablespoons olive oil
- 1 tablespoon hot sauce
- 1 tablespoon sweet paprika
- 1 tablespoon tomato puree
- Salt and black pepper to the taste
- ½ bunch cilantro, chopped
- 2 garlic cloves, minced

Directions:
In a pan that fits the air fryer, mix all the ingredients, toss, introduce in the fryer and cook at 380 degrees F for 20 minutes. Divide the stew into bowls and serve for lunch.

Nutrition: calories 183, fat 4, fiber 2, carbs 4, protein 12

Lamb and Veggies
*Prep time: 5 minutes | **Cooking time:** 30 minutes | **Servings:** 4*

Ingredients:

- 1 pound lamb shoulder, trimmed and cubed
- 2 tablespoons olive oil
- 3 garlic cloves, minced
- 4 baby leeks, halved
- 1 cup okra
- 20 ounces canned tomatoes, peeled and chopped
- Salt and black pepper to the taste
- 2 tablespoons tarragon, chopped

Directions:

Heat up a pan that fits your air fryer with the oil over medium-high heat, add the lamb, garlic, salt and pepper, toss and brown for 5 minutes. Add the remaining ingredients except the tarragon, toss, introduce the pan in the fryer and cook at 400 degrees F for 25 minutes. Divide everything into bowls and serve for lunch.

Nutrition: calories 235, fat 12, fiber 4, carbs 5, protein 15

Pork and Brussels Sprouts Stew
*Prep time: 5 minutes | **Cooking time:** 25 minutes | **Servings:** 4*

Ingredients:

- 2 tablespoons olive oil
- 2 tomatoes, cubed
- 2 garlic cloves, minced
- ½ pound Brussels sprouts, halved
- 1 pound pork stew meat, cubed
- ¼ cup veggie stock
- ¼ cup tomato puree
- Salt and black pepper to the taste
- 1 tablespoon chives, chopped

Directions:

Heat up a pan that fits the air fryer with the oil over medium-high heat, add the meat, garlic, salt and pepper, stir and brown for 5 minutes. Add all the other ingredients except the chives, toss, introduce in the fryer and cook at 380 degrees F for 20 minutes. Divide the stew into bowls and serve with chives sprinkled on top.

Nutrition: calories 200, fat 6, fiber 2, carbs 4, protein 13

Italian Beef
Prep time: 5 minutes | *Cooking time:* 25 minutes | *Servings:* 4

Ingredients:

- 1 and ½ pounds beef stew meat, cubed
- ½ cup green onions, chopped
- 3 tablespoons butter, melted
- ½ cup celery, chopped
- 1 garlic clove, minced
- ½ teaspoon Italian seasoning
- 15 ounces canned tomatoes, chopped
- Salt and black pepper to the taste

Directions:

Heat up a pan that fits your air fryer with the butter over medium heat, add the meat, toss and brown for 5 minutes. Add the rest of the ingredients, toss, introduce the pan in the fryer and cook at 390 degrees F for 20 minutes. Divide into bowls and serve for lunch.

Nutrition: calories 224, fat 14, fiber 3, carbs 5, protein 14

Ketogenic Air Fryer Side Dish Recipes

Baked Cauliflower Rice
Prep time: 5 minutes | Cooking time: 20 minutes | Servings: 4

Ingredients:

- 1 big cauliflower, florets separated and riced
- 1 and ½ cups chicken stock
- 1 tablespoon olive oil
- Salt and black pepper to the taste
- ½ teaspoon turmeric powder

Directions:

In a pan that fits the air fryer, combine the cauliflower with the oil and the rest of the ingredients, toss, introduce in the air fryer and cook at 360 degrees F for 20 minutes. Divide between plates and serve as a side dish.

Nutrition: calories 193, fat 5, fiber 2, carbs 4, protein 6

Cheese Cauliflower Bake
Prep time: 5 minutes | Cooking time: 20 minutes | Servings: 2

Ingredients:

- 1 cup heavy whipping cream
- 2 tablespoons basil pesto
- Salt and black pepper to the taste
- Juice of ½ lemon
- 1 pound cauliflower, florets separated
- 4 ounces cherry tomatoes, halved
- 3 tablespoons ghee, melted
- 7 ounces cheddar cheese, grated

Directions:

Grease a baking pan that fits the air fryer with the ghee. Add the cauliflower, lemon juice, salt, pepper, the pesto and the cream and toss gently. Add the tomatoes, sprinkle the cheese on top, introduce the pan in the fryer and cook at 380 degrees F for 20 minutes. Divide between plates and serve as a side dish.

Nutrition: calories 200, fat 7, fiber 2, carbs 4, protein 7

Creamy Brussels Sprouts
Prep time: 5 minutes | Cooking time: 20 minutes | Servings: 4

Ingredients:

- 1 pound Brussels sprouts, trimmed and halved
- Salt and black pepper to the taste
- 2 tablespoons ghee, melted
- ½ cup coconut cream
- 2 tablespoons garlic, minced
- 1 tablespoon chives, chopped

Directions:

In your air fryer, mix the sprouts with the rest of the ingredients except the chives, toss well, introduce in the air fryer and cook them at 370 degrees F for 20 minutes. Divide the Brussels sprouts between plates, sprinkle the chives on top and serve as a side dish.

Nutrition: calories 194, fat 6, fiber 2, carbs 4, protein 8

Mustard Broccoli and Cauliflower
Prep time: 5 minutes | Cooking time: 20 minutes | Servings: 4

Ingredients:

- 15 ounces broccoli florets
- 10 ounces cauliflower florets
- 1 leek, chopped
- 2 spring onions, chopped
- Salt and black pepper to the taste
- 2 ounces butter, melted
- 2 tablespoons mustard
- 1 cup sour cream
- 5 ounces mozzarella cheese, shredded

Directions:

In a baking pan that fits the air fryer, add the butter and spread it well. Add the broccoli, cauliflower and the rest of the ingredients except the mozzarella and toss. Sprinkle the cheese on top, introduce the pan in the air fryer and cook at 380 degrees F for 20 minutes. Divide between plates and serve as a side dish.

Nutrition: calories 242, fat 13, fiber 2, carbs 4, protein 8

Mushroom Risotto
Prep time: 5 minutes | Cooking time: 20 minutes | Servings: 4

Ingredients:
- 1 pound white mushrooms, sliced
- ¼ cup mozzarella, shredded
- 1 cauliflower head, florets separated and riced
- 1 cup chicken stock
- 1 tablespoon thyme, chopped
- 1 teaspoon Italian seasoning
- A pinch of salt and black pepper
- 2 tablespoons olive oil

Directions:
Heat up a pan that fits the air fryer with the oil over medium heat, add the cauliflower rice and the mushrooms, toss and cook for a couple of minutes. Add the rest of the ingredients except the thyme, toss, put the pan in the air fryer and cook at 360 degrees F for 20 minutes. Divide the risotto between plates and serve with thyme sprinkled on top

Nutrition: calories 204, fat 12, fiber 3, carbs 4, protein 8

Mustard Spinach Side Salad
Prep time: 5 minutes | Cooking time: 10 minutes | Servings: 4

Ingredients:
- 1 pound baby spinach
- Salt and black pepper to the taste
- 1 tablespoon mustard
- Cooking spray
- ¼ cup apple cider vinegar
- 1 tablespoon chives, chopped

Directions:
Grease a pan that fits your air fryer with cooking spray, combine all the ingredients, introduce the pan in the fryer and cook at 350 degrees F for 10 minutes. Divide between plates and serve as a side dish.

Nutrition: calories 160, fat 3, fiber 2, carbs 4, protein 6

Cauliflower Hash Browns
Prep time: 5 minutes | Cooking time: 15 minutes | Servings: 4

Ingredients:
- 1 pound cauliflower florets, roughly grated
- 3 eggs, whisked
- 3 tablespoons butter, melted
- Salt and black pepper to the taste
- 1 tablespoon sweet paprika

Directions:
Heat up a pan that fits the air fryer with the butter over high heat, add the cauliflower and brown for 5 minutes. Add whisked eggs, salt, pepper and the paprika, toss, introduce the pan in the fryer and cook at 400 degrees F for 10 minutes. Divide between plates and serve.

Nutrition: calories 153, fat 5, fiber 2, carbs 5, protein 5

Roasted Cauliflower Mash
Prep time: 5 minutes | Cooking time: 20 minutes | Servings: 4

Ingredients:
- 2 pounds cauliflower florets
- 1 teaspoon olive oil
- 3 ounces parmesan, grated
- 4 ounces butter, soft
- Juice of ½ lemon
- Zest of ½ lemon, grated
- Salt and black pepper to the taste

Directions:
Preheated you air fryer at 380 degrees F, add the basket inside, add the cauliflower, also add the oil, rub well and cook for 20 minutes. Transfer the cauliflower to a bowl, mash well, add the rest of the ingredients, stir really well, divide between plates and serve as a side dish.

Nutrition: calories 174, fat 5, fiber 2, carbs 5, protein 8

Roasted Fennel Mix
Prep time: 5 minutes | Cooking time: 15 minutes | Servings: 4

Ingredients:

- 1 pound fennel, cut into small wedges
- A pinch of salt and black pepper
- 3 tablespoons olive oil
- Salt and black pepper to the taste
- Juice of ½ lemon
- 2 tablespoons sunflower seeds

Directions:

In a bowl, mix the fennel wedges with all the ingredients except the sunflower seeds, put them in your air fryer's basket and cook at 400 degrees F for 15 minutes. Divide the fennel between plates, sprinkle the sunflower seeds on top, and serve as a side dish.

Nutrition: calories 152, fat 4, fiber 2, carbs 4, protein 7

Mini Peppers Mix
Prep time: 5 minutes | Cooking time: 20 minutes | Servings: 4

Ingredients:

- 8 ounces mini bell peppers, halved
- 1 tablespoon olive oil
- 1 tablespoon cilantro, chopped
- 8 ounces cream cheese, soft
- 1 cup cheddar cheese, shredded
- Salt and black pepper to the taste

Directions:

Grease a baking dish that fits the air fryer with the oil and arrange the bell peppers inside. In a bowl, mix all the ingredients, whisk well, spread over the bell peppers, introduce the dish in the air fryer and cook at 370 degrees F for 20 minutes. Divide the peppers between plates and serve as a side dish.

Nutrition: calories 200, fat 8, fiber 2, carbs 5, protein 8

Warm Coleslaw
Prep time: 5 minutes | Cooking time: 20 minutes | Servings: 4

Ingredients:
- 1 green cabbage head, shredded
- Juice of ½ lemon
- A pinch of salt and black pepper
- ½ cup coconut cream
- ½ teaspoon fennel seeds
- 1 tablespoon mustard

Directions:
In a pan that fits the air fryer, combine the cabbage with the rest of the ingredients, toss, introduce the pan in the machine and cook at 350 degrees F for 20 minutes. Divide between plates and serve right away as a side dish.

Nutrition: calories 202, fat 9, fiber 3, carbs 4, protein 7

Simple Roasted Cabbage
Prep time: 4 minutes | Cooking time: 25 minutes | Servings: 4

Ingredients:
- 1 green cabbage head, shredded and cut into large wedges
- 2 tablespoons olive oil
- 1 tablespoon cilantro, chopped
- 1 tablespoon lemon juice
- A pinch of salt and black pepper

Directions:
Preheat your air fryer at 370 degrees F, add the cabbage wedges mixed with all the ingredients in the basket and cook for 25 minutes. Divide between plates and serve as a side dish.

Nutrition: calories 185, fat 6, fiber 3, carbs 5, protein 4

Rutabaga Fries
Prep time: 5 minutes | Cooking time: 20 minutes | Servings: 4

Ingredients:
- 15 ounces rutabaga, cut into fries
- 4 tablespoons olive oil
- 1 teaspoon chili powder
- A pinch of salt and black pepper

Directions:
In a bowl, mix the rutabaga fries with all the other ingredients, toss and put them in your air fryer's basket. Cook at 400 degrees F for 20 minutes, divide between plates and serve as a side dish.

Nutrition: calories 176, fat 8, fiber 2, carbs 4, protein 4

Eggplant Hash
Prep time: 5 minutes | Cooking time: 15 minutes | Servings: 4

Ingredients:
- 2 tablespoons olive oil
- 2 eggplants, roughly cubed
- 8 ounces mozzarella cheese, shredded
- 3 spring onions, chopped
- Juice of 1 lime
- 2 tablespoons butter, melted
- 4 eggs, whisked

Directions:
Heat up a pan that fits the air fryer with the oil and the butter over medium-high heat, add the spring onions and the eggplants, stir and cook for 5 minutes. Add the eggs and lime juice and stir well. Sprinkle the cheese on top, introduce the pan in the fryer and cook at 380 degrees F for 10 minutes. Divide between plates and serve as a side dish.

Nutrition: calories 212, fat 9, fiber 2, carbs 4, protein 12

Roasted Veggies

Prep time: 5 minutes | *Cooking time:* 20 minutes | *Servings:* 4

Ingredients:

- 1 pound Brussels sprouts, halved
- 1 tablespoon olive oil
- 8 ounces brown mushrooms, halved
- 8 ounces cherry tomatoes, halved
- 1 teaspoon rosemary, dried
- A pinch of salt and black pepper
- Juice of 1 lime

Directions:

In a bowl, mix all the ingredients, toss, put them in your air fryer's basket, cook at 380 degrees F for 20 minutes, divide between plates and serve as a side dish.

Nutrition: calories 163, fat 4, fiber 2, carbs 4, protein 8

Cabbage Sauté

Prep time: 5 minutes | *Cooking time:* 20 minutes | *Servings:* 4

Ingredients:

- 2 ounces butter, melted
- 1 green cabbage head, shredded
- 1 and ½ cups heavy cream
- ¼ cup parsley, chopped
- 1 tablespoon sweet paprika
- 1 teaspoon lemon zest, grated

Directions:

Heat up a pan that fits the air fryer with the butter, add the cabbage and sauté for 5 minutes. Add the remaining ingredients, toss, put the pan in the air fryer and cook at 380 degrees F for 15 minutes. Divide between plates and serve as a side dish.

Nutrition: calories 174, fat 4, fiber 3, carbs 5, protein 8

Green Beans and Sauce
Prep time: 5 minutes | Cooking time: 20 minutes | Servings: 4

Ingredients:
- 10 ounces green beans, trimmed
- A pinch of salt and black pepper
- 3 ounces butter, melted
- 1 cup coconut cream
- Zest of ½ lemon, grated
- ¼ cup parsley, chopped
- 2 garlic cloves, minced

Directions:
In a bowl, the butter with all the ingredients except the green beans and whisk really well. Put the green beans in a pan that fits the air fryer, drizzle the buttery sauce all over, introduce the pan in the machine and cook at 370 degrees F for 20 minutes. Divide between plates and serve as a side dish.

Nutrition: calories 200, fat 9, fiber 2, carbs 4, protein 9

Curry Cabbage
Prep time: 5 minutes | Cooking time: 20 minutes | Servings: 4

Ingredients:
- 30 ounces green cabbage, shredded
- 1 tablespoon red curry paste
- 3 tablespoons coconut oil, melted
- A pinch of salt and black pepper

Directions:
In a pan that fits the air fryer, combine the cabbage with the rest of the ingredients, toss, introduce the pan in the machine and cook at 380 degrees F for 20 minutes. Divide between plates and serve as a side dish.

Nutrition: calories 180, fat 14, fiber 4, carbs 6, protein 8

Broccoli Mash
Prep time: 5 minutes | Cooking time: 20 minutes | Servings: 4

Ingredients:
- 20 ounces broccoli florets
- A drizzle of olive oil
- 4 tablespoons basil, chopped
- 3 ounces butter, melted
- 1 garlic clove, minced
- A pinch of salt and black pepper

Directions:
In a bowl, mix the broccoli with the oil, salt and pepper, toss and transfer to your air fryer's basket. Cook at 380 degrees F for 20 minutes, cool the broccoli down and put it in a blender. Add the rest of the ingredients, pulse, divide the mash between plates and serve as a side dish.

Nutrition: calories 200, fat 14, fiber 3, carbs 6, protein 7

Zucchinis and Walnuts Mix
Prep time: 5 minutes | Cooking time: 20 minutes | Servings: 4

Ingredients:
- 1 pound zucchinis, sliced
- 1 tablespoon olive oil
- Salt and white pepper to the taste
- 4 ounces arugula leaves
- ¼ cup chives, chopped
- 1 cup walnuts, chopped

Directions:
In a pan that fits the air fryer, combine all the ingredients except the arugula and walnuts, toss, put the pan in the machine and cook at 360 degrees F for 20 minutes. Transfer this to a salad bowl, add the arugula and the walnuts, toss and serve as a side salad.

Nutrition: calories 170, fat 4, fiber 1, carbs 4, protein 5

Dill Red Cabbage
Prep time: 5 minutes | Cooking time: 20 minutes | Servings: 4

Ingredients:

- 30 ounces red cabbage, shredded
- 4 ounces butter, melted
- A pinch of salt and black pepper
- 1 teaspoon cinnamon powder
- 1 tablespoon red wine vinegar
- 2 tablespoons dill, chopped

Directions:

In a pan that fits your air fryer, mix the cabbage with the rest of the ingredients, toss, put the pan in the machine and cook at 390 degrees F for 20 minutes. Divide between plates and serve as a side dish.

Nutrition: calories 201, fat 17, fiber 2, carbs 5, protein 5

Crispy Brussels Sprouts
Prep time: 5 minutes | Cooking time: 15 minutes | Servings: 4

Ingredients:

- 1 pound Brussels sprouts, trimmed and shredded
- ½ cup olive oil
- Juice of 1 lemon
- Zest of 1 lemon, grated
- A pinch of salt and black pepper
- ¼ cup almonds, toasted and chopped
- ½ teaspoon cumin, crushed
- 1 teaspoon chili paste

Directions:

In a pan that fits the air fryer, combine the Brussels sprouts with all the other ingredients, toss, put the pan in the fryer and cook at 390 degrees F for 15 minutes. Divide between plates and serve as a side dish.

Nutrition: calories 200, fat 9, fiber 2, carbs 6, protein 9

Goat Cheese Cauliflower
Prep time: 5 minutes | Cooking time: 20 minutes | Servings: 4

Ingredients:
- 8 cups cauliflower florets, roughly chopped
- 4 bacon strips, chopped
- Salt and black pepper to the taste
- ½ cup spring onions, chopped
- 1 tablespoon garlic, minced
- 10 ounces goat cheese, crumbled
- ¼ cup soft cream cheese
- Cooking spray

Directions:
Grease a baking pan that fits the air fryer with the cooking spray and mix all the ingredients except the goat cheese into the pan. Sprinkle the cheese on top, introduce the pan in the machine and cook at 400 degrees F for 20 minutes. Divide between plates and serve as a side dish.

Nutrition: calories 203, fat 13, fiber 2, carbs 5, protein 9

Spiced Cauliflower
Prep time: 5 minutes | Cooking time: 15 minutes | Servings: 4

Ingredients:
- 1 cauliflower head, florets separated
- 1 tablespoon butter, melted
- A pinch of salt and black pepper
- 1 tablespoon olive oil
- ¼ teaspoon turmeric powder
- ½ teaspoon cumin, ground
- ¼ teaspoon cinnamon powder
- ¼ teaspoon cloves, ground

Directions:
In a bowl, mix cauliflower florets with the rest of the ingredients and toss. Put the cauliflower in your air fryer's basket and cook at 390 degrees F for 15 minutes. Divide between plates and serve as a side dish.

Nutrition: calories 182, fat 8, fiber 2, carbs 4, protein 8

Cauliflower and Kale Mash

Prep time: 5 minutes | *Cooking time:* 20 minutes | *Servings:* 4

Ingredients:

- 1 cauliflower head, florets separated
- 4 teaspoons butter, melted
- 4 garlic cloves, minced
- 3 cups kale, chopped
- 2 scallions, chopped
- A pinch of salt and black pepper
- 1/3 cup coconut cream
- 1 tablespoon parsley, chopped

Directions:

In a pan that fits the air fryer, combine the cauliflower with the butter, garlic, scallions, salt, pepper and the cream, toss, introduce the pan in the machine and cook at 380 degrees F for 20 minutes. Mash the mix well, add the remaining ingredients, whisk, divide between plates and serve.

Nutrition: calories 198, fat 9, fiber 2, carbs 6, protein 8

Mexican Cauliflower Bake

Prep time: 5 minutes | *Cooking time:* 20 minutes | *Servings:* 4

Ingredients:

- 2 cups cauliflower florets, roughly chopped
- 1 tablespoon olive oil
- Salt and black pepper to the taste
- 4 garlic cloves, minced
- 1 red chili pepper, chopped
- 2 tomatoes, cubed
- 1 teaspoon cumin powder
- ½ teaspoon chili powder
- 1 tablespoon coriander, chopped
- 1 avocado, peeled, pitted and sliced
- 1 tablespoon lime juice

Directions:

In a pan that fits the air fryer, combine the cauliflower with the other ingredients except the coriander, avocado and lime juice, toss, introduce the pan in the machine and cook at 380 degrees F for 20 minutes. Divide between plates, top each serving with coriander, avocado and lime juice and serve as a side dish.

Nutrition: calories 187, fat 8, fiber 2, carbs 5, protein 7

Coconut Cauliflower Risotto

Prep time: 5 minutes | Cooking time: 20 minutes | Servings: 4

Ingredients:

- 2 cups cauliflower rice
- 1 cup coconut milk
- 2 tablespoons coconut oil, melted
- 1 tablespoon cilantro, chopped
- 1 tablespoon olive oil
- 1 teaspoon lime zest, grated
- 2 tablespoons parmesan, grated

Directions:

In a pan that fits your air fryer, mix all the ingredients, stir, introduce in the fryer and cook at 360 degrees F for 20 minutes. Divide between plates and serve as a side dish.

Nutrition: calories 193, fat 4, fiber 3, carbs 5, protein 6

Risotto and Sun-dried Tomatoes

Prep time: 5 minutes | Cooking time: 20 minutes | Servings: 6

Ingredients:

- 2 tablespoons butter, melted
- 1 pound cauliflower, riced
- 2 garlic cloves, minced
- ½ cup chicken stock
- 1 cup heavy cream
- 1 cup parmesan, grated
- 3 tablespoons sun-dried tomatoes
- ½ teaspoon nutmeg, ground

Directions:

Heat up a pan that fits your air fryer with the butter over medium heat, add cauliflower rice, stir and cook for 2 minutes. Add the rest of the ingredients, toss, introduce the pan in the fryer and cook at 360 degrees F for 20 minutes. Divide between plates and serve as a side dish.

Nutrition: calories 193, fat 8, fiber 2, carbs 5, protein 9

Mashed Celeriac
Prep time: 5 *minutes* | *Cooking time:* 20 *minutes* | *Servings:* 4

Ingredients:
- 14 ounces celeriac, chopped
- 1 cup cauliflower florets
- Salt and black pepper to the taste
- 2 garlic cloves, minced
- 1/3 cup heavy cream
- 4 ounces butter, melted
- 1 tablespoon chives, chopped
- Zest of 1 lemon, grated

Directions:
In a pan that fits your air fryer, mix all the ingredients except the chives and the cream, stir, introduce the pan in the machine and cook at 360 degrees F for 20 minutes. Mash the mix, add the rest of the ingredients, whisk well, divide between plates and serve as a side dish.

Nutrition: calories 201, fat 9, fiber 2, carbs 6, protein 9

Balsamic Zucchinis and Cheese
Prep time: 5 *minutes* | *Cooking time:* 20 *minutes* | *Servings:* 4

Ingredients:
- 2 pounds zucchinis, sliced
- 2 ounces feta cheese, crumbled
- 1 tablespoon parsley, chopped
- ¼ cup olive oil
- 2 tablespoons balsamic vinegar
- 1 teaspoon thyme, dried
- A pinch of salt and black pepper

Directions:
In a pan that fits your air fryer, mix the zucchini slices with the other ingredients except the cheese and toss. Sprinkle the cheese on top, introduce the pan in the fryer and cook at 400 degrees F for 20 minutes. Divide between plates and serve as a side dish.

Nutrition: calories 203, fat 9, fiber 3, carbs 6, protein 5

Zucchini Noodles and Sauce

Prep time: 5 minutes | Cooking time: 15 minutes | Servings: 4

Ingredients:

- 4 zucchinis, cut with a spiralizer
- 1 tablespoon olive oil
- 4 garlic cloves, minced
- 1 and ½ cups tomatoes, crushed
- Salt and black pepper to the taste
- 1 tablespoon basil, chopped
- ¼ cup green onions, chopped

Directions:

In a pan that fits your air fryer, mix zucchini noodles with the other ingredients, toss, introduce in the fryer and cook at 380 degrees F for 15 minutes. Divide between plates and serve as a side dish.

Nutrition: calories 194, fat 7, fiber 2, carbs 4, protein 9

Zucchini Gratin

Prep time: 5 minutes | Cooking time: 25 minutes | Servings: 4

Ingredients:

- 4 cups zucchinis, sliced
- 1 and ½ cups mozzarella, shredded
- 2 tablespoons butter, melted
- ½ teaspoon garlic powder
- ½ cup coconut cream
- ½ tablespoon parsley, chopped

Directions:

In a baking pan that fits the air fryer, mix all the ingredients except the mozzarella and the parsley, and toss. Sprinkle the mozzarella and parsley, introduce in the air fryer and cook at 370 degrees F for 25 minutes. Divide between plates and serve as a side dish.

Nutrition: calories 220, fat 14, fiber 2, carbs 5, protein 9

Artichokes and Cauliflower
Prep time: 5 minutes | Cooking time: 20 minutes | Servings: 4

Ingredients:

- 1 tablespoon olive oil
- 1 cup cauliflower florets
- 2 garlic cloves, minced
- ½ cup chicken stock
- 15 ounces canned artichoke hearts, chopped
- 1 tablespoon parmesan, grated
- 1 and ½ tablespoons parsley, chopped
- Salt and black pepper to the taste

Directions:

In a pan that fits your air fryer, mix all the ingredients except the parmesan and toss. Sprinkle the parmesan on top, introduce the pan in the air fryer and cook at 380 degrees F for 20 minutes. Divide between plates and serve as a side dish.

Nutrition: calories 195, fat 6, fiber 2, carbs 4, protein 8

Minty Summer Squash
Prep time: 5 minutes | Cooking time: 25 minutes | Servings: 4

Ingredients:

- 4 summer squash, cut into wedges
- ¼ cup olive oil
- ¼ cup lemon juice
- ½ cup mint, chopped
- 1 cup mozzarella, shredded
- Salt and black pepper to the taste

Directions:

In a pan that fits your air fryer, mix the squash with the rest of the ingredients, toss, introduce the pan in the air fryer and cook at 370 degrees F for 25 minutes. Divide between plates and serve as a side dish.

Nutrition: calories 201, fat 7, fiber 2, carbs 4, protein 9

Pesto Zucchini Pasta
Prep time: 5 minutes | *Cooking time:* 15 minutes | *Servings:* 4

Ingredients:

- 2 cups zucchinis, cut with a spiralizer
- Salt and black pepper to the taste
- 1 tablespoon olive oil
- ½ cup coconut cream
- 4 ounces mozzarella, shredded
- ¼ cup basil pesto

Directions:

In a pan that fits your air fryer, mix the zucchini noodles with the pesto and the rest of the ingredients, toss, introduce the pan in the fryer and cook at 370 degrees F for 15 minutes. Divide between plates and serve as a side dish.

Nutrition: calories 200, fat 8, fiber 2, carbs 4, protein 10

Hot Green Beans
Prep time: 5 minutes | *Cooking time:* 20 minutes | *Servings:* 4

Ingredients:

- 6 cups green beans, trimmed
- 2 tablespoons olive oil
- 1 tablespoon hot paprika
- A pinch of salt and black pepper

Directions:

In a bowl, mix the green beans with the other ingredients, toss, put them in the air fryer's basket and cook at 370 degrees F for 20 minutes. Divide between plates and serve as a side dish.

Nutrition: calories 120, fat 5, fiber 1, carbs 4, protein 2

Balsamic Asparagus
Prep time: 5 minutes | Cooking time: 20 minutes | Servings: 4

Ingredients:

- 1 pound asparagus stalks
- Salt and black pepper to the taste
- ¼ cup olive oil+ 1 teaspoon
- 1 tablespoon smoked paprika
- 2 tablespoons balsamic vinegar
- 1 tablespoon lime juice

Directions:

In a bowl, mix the asparagus with salt, pepper and 1 teaspoon oil, toss, transfer to your air fryer's basket and cook at 370 degrees F for 20 minutes. Meanwhile, in a bowl, mix all the other ingredients and whisk them well. Divide the asparagus between plates, drizzle the balsamic vinaigrette all over and serve as a side dish.

Nutrition: calories 187, fat 6, fiber 2, carbs 4, protein 9

Garlic Asparagus
Prep time: 5 minutes | Cooking time: 15 minutes | Servings: 4

Ingredients:

- 1 bunch asparagus, trimmed
- Salt and black pepper to the taste
- 4 tablespoons olive oil
- 4 garlic cloves, minced
- Juice of ½ lemon
- 3 tablespoons parmesan, grated

Directions:

In a bowl, mix the asparagus with all the ingredients except the parmesan, toss, transfer it to your air fryer's basket and cook at 400 degrees F for 15 minutes. Divide between plates, sprinkle the parmesan on top and serve as a side dish.

Nutrition: calories 173, fat 12, fiber 2, carbs 5, protein 7

Collard Greens Sauté

Prep time: 5 minutes | *Cooking time:* 15 minutes | *Servings:* 4

Ingredients:
- 1 pound collard greens
- ¼ cup cherry tomatoes, halved
- 1 tablespoon balsamic vinegar
- A pinch of salt and black pepper
- 2 tablespoons chicken stock

Directions:
In a pan that fits your air fryer, mix the collard greens with the other ingredients, toss gently, introduce in the air fryer and cook at 360 degrees F for 15 minutes. Divide between plates and serve as a side dish.

Nutrition: calories 121, fat 3, fiber 4, carbs 6, protein 5

Hot Zucchini Spaghetti

Prep time: 5 minutes | *Cooking time:* 15 minutes | *Servings:* 4

Ingredients:
- 1 pound zucchinis, cut with a spiralizer
- ¼ cup olive oil
- Salt and black pepper to the taste
- 6 garlic cloves, minced
- ½ teaspoon red pepper flakes
- 1 cup parmesan, grated
- ¼ cup parsley, chopped

Directions:
In a pan that fits your air fryer, mix all the ingredients, toss, introduce in the fryer and cook at 370 degrees F for 15 minutes. Divide between plates and serve as a side dish.

Nutrition: calories 200, fat 6, fiber 3, carbs 4, protein 5

Garlicky Zucchini Noodles

Prep time: 5 minutes | Cooking time: 15 minutes | Servings: 4

Ingredients:

- 1 pound zucchinis, cut with a spiralizer
- 2 tomatoes, cubed
- 3 tablespoons butter, melted
- 4 garlic cloves, minced
- 3 tablespoons parsley, chopped
- Salt and black pepper to the taste

Directions:

In a pan that fits your air fryer, mix all the ingredients, toss, introduce in the fryer and cook at 350 degrees F for 15 minutes. Divide between plates and serve as a side dish.

Nutrition: calories 170, fat 6, fiber 2, carbs 5, protein 6

Cherry Tomatoes and Scallions Mix

Prep time: 5 minutes | Cooking time: 15 minutes | Servings: 4

Ingredients:

- 1 tablespoon ghee, melted
- 2 cups cherry tomatoes, halved
- 3 tablespoons scallions, chopped
- 1 teaspoon lemon zest, grated
- 2 tablespoons parsley, chopped
- ¼ cup parmesan, grated

Directions:

In a pan that fits the air fryer, combine all the ingredients except the parmesan, and toss. Sprinkle the parmesan on top, introduce the pan in the machine and cook at 360 degrees F for 10 minutes. Divide between plates and serve.

Nutrition: calories 141, fat 6, fiber 2, carbs 4, protein 7

Creamy Fennel
Prep time: 5 minutes | Cooking time: 12 minutes | Servings: 4

Ingredients:
- 2 big fennel bulbs, sliced
- 2 tablespoons butter, melted
- Salt and black pepper to the taste
- ½ cup coconut cream

Directions:
In a pan that fits the air fryer, combine all the ingredients, toss, introduce in the machine and cook at 370 degrees F for 12 minutes. Divide between plates and serve as a side dish.

Nutrition: calories 151, fat 3, fiber 2, carbs 4, protein 6

Cream Cheese Zucchini
Prep time: 5 minutes | Cooking time: 15 minutes | Servings: 4

Ingredients:
- 1 pound zucchinis, cut into wedges
- 1 cup cream cheese, soft
- 1 green onion, sliced
- 1 teaspoon garlic powder
- 2 tablespoons basil, chopped
- A pinch of salt and black pepper
- 1 tablespoon butter, melted

Directions:
In a pan that fits your air fryer, mix the zucchinis with all the other ingredients, toss, introduce in the air fryer and cook at 370 degrees F for 15 minutes. Divide between plates and serve as a side dish.

Nutrition: calories 129, fat 6, fiber 2, carbs 5, protein 8

Parmesan Zucchini Rounds
Prep time: 5 minutes | Cooking time: 20 minutes | Servings: 4

Ingredients:
- 4 zucchinis, sliced
- 1 egg, whisked
- 1 egg white, whisked
- 1 and ½ cups parmesan, grated
- ¼ cup parsley, chopped
- ½ teaspoon garlic powder
- Cooking spray

Directions:
In a bowl, mix the egg with egg whites, parmesan, parsley and garlic powder and whisk. Dredge each zucchini slice in this mix, place them all in your air fryer's basket, grease them with cooking spray and cook at 370 degrees F for 20 minutes. Divide between plates and serve as a side dish.

Nutrition: calories 183, fat 6, fiber 2, carbs 3, protein 8

Kale and Walnuts
Prep time: 5 minutes | Cooking time: 15 minutes | Servings: 4

Ingredients:
- 1 tablespoon butter, melted
- ½ cup almond milk
- Salt and black pepper to the taste
- 3 garlic cloves
- 10 cups kale, roughly chopped
- ¼ teaspoon nutmeg, ground
- 1/3 cup parmesan, grated
- ¼ cup walnuts, chopped

Directions:
In a pan that fits the air fryer, combine all the ingredients, toss, introduce the pan in the machine and cook at 360 degrees F for 15 minutes. Divide between plates and serve.

Nutrition: calories 160, fat 7, fiber 2, carbs 4, protein 5

Kale and Pine Nuts
Prep time: 5 minutes | Cooking time: 15 minutes | Servings: 4

Ingredients:
- 10 cups kale, torn
- 2 tablespoons olive oil
- Salt and black pepper to the taste
- 2 tablespoons lemon zest, grated
- 1 tablespoon lemon juice
- 1/3 cup pine nuts

Directions:
In a pan that fits the air fryer, combine all the ingredients, toss, introduce the pan in the machine and cook at 380 degrees F for 15 minutes. Divide between plates and serve as a side dish.

Nutrition: calories 121, fat 9, fiber 2, carbs 4, protein 5

Bok Choy and Butter Sauce
Prep time: 5 minutes | Cooking time: 15 minutes | Servings: 4

Ingredients:
- 2 tablespoons chicken stock
- 1 tablespoon olive oil
- 2 bok choy heads, trimmed and cut into strips
- 1 tablespoon butter, melted
- A pinch of salt and black pepper
- 1 teaspoon lemon juice

Directions:
In a pan that fits your air fryer, mix all the ingredients, toss, introduce the pan in the air fryer and cook at 380 degrees F for 15 minutes. Divide between plates and serve as a side dish.

Nutrition: calories 141, fat 3, fiber 2, carbs 4, protein 3

Balsamic Cabbage
Prep time: 10 minutes | Cooking time: 15 minutes | Servings: 4

Ingredients:
- 4 garlic cloves, minced
- 1 tablespoon olive oil
- 6 cups red cabbage, shredded
- 1 tablespoon balsamic vinegar
- Salt and black pepper to the taste

Directions:
In a pan that fits the air fryer, combine all the ingredients, toss, introduce the pan in the air fryer and cook at 380 degrees F for 15 minutes. Divide between plates and serve as a side dish.

Nutrition: calories 151, fat 2, fiber 3, carbs 5, protein 5

Radishes and Sesame Seeds
Prep time: 5 minutes | Cooking time: 15 minutes | Servings: 4

Ingredients:
- 20 radishes, halved
- 1 tablespoon olive oil
- 2 spring onions, chopped
- 3 green onions, chopped
- Salt and black pepper to the taste
- 3 teaspoons black sesame seeds
- 2 tablespoons olive oil

Directions:
In a bowl, mix all the ingredients and toss well. Put the radishes in your air fryer's basket, cook at 400 degrees F for 15 minutes, divide between plates and serve as a side dish.

Nutrition: calories 150, fat 4, fiber 2, carbs 3, protein 5

Herbed Radish Sauté
Prep time: 5 minutes | Cooking time: 15 minutes | Servings: 4

Ingredients:
- 2 bunches red radishes, halved
- 1 tablespoon olive oil
- 2 tablespoons balsamic vinegar
- 2 tablespoons parsley, chopped
- Salt and black pepper to the taste

Directions:
In a bowl, mix the radishes with the remaining ingredients except the parsley, toss and put them in your air fryer's basket. Cook at 400 degrees F for 15 minutes, divide between plates, sprinkle the parsley on top and serve as a side dish.

Nutrition: calories 180, fat 4, fiber 2, carbs 3, protein 5

Radishes and Cabbage Mix
Prep time: 5 minutes | Cooking time: 15 minutes | Servings: 4

Ingredients:
- 6 cups green cabbage, shredded
- 6 radishes, sliced
- ½ cup celery leaves, chopped
- ¼ cup green onions, chopped
- 2 tablespoons balsamic vinegar
- 1 teaspoon lemon juice
- 3 tablespoons olive oil
- ½ teaspoon hot paprika

Directions:
In your air fryer's pan, combine all the ingredients and toss well. Introduce the pan in the fryer and cook at 380 degrees F for 15 minutes. Divide between plates and serve as a side dish.

Nutrition: calories 130, fat 4, fiber 3, carbs 4, protein 7

Chives Radishes
Prep time: 5 minutes | Cooking time: 15 minutes | Servings: 4

Ingredients:
- 20 radishes, halved
- 1 teaspoon chives, chopped
- 1 tablespoon garlic, minced
- Salt and black pepper to the taste
- 2 tablespoons olive oil

Directions:
In your air fryer's pan, combine all the ingredients and toss. Introduce the pan in the machine and cook at 370 degrees F for 15 minutes. Divide between plates and serve as a side dish.

Nutrition: calories 160, fat 2, fiber 3, carbs 4, protein 6

Roasted Tomatoes
Prep time: 5 minutes | Cooking time: 15 minutes | Servings: 4

Ingredients:
- 4 tomatoes, halved
- ½ teaspoon smoked paprika
- ½ teaspoon garlic powder
- ½ teaspoon onion powder
- ½ teaspoon oregano, dried
- 1 tablespoon basil, chopped
- ½ cup parmesan, grated
- Cooking spray

Directions:
In a bowl, mix all the ingredients except the cooking spray and the parmesan. Arrange the tomatoes in your air fryer's pan, sprinkle the parmesan on top and grease with cooking spray. Cook at 370 degrees F for 15 minutes, divide between plates and serve.

Nutrition: calories 200, fat 7, fiber 2, carbs 4, protein 6

Chili Endives

Prep time: 5 minutes | Cooking time: 20 minutes | Servings: 4

Ingredients:

- 2 scallions, chopped
- 3 garlic cloves, minced
- 1 tablespoon olive oil
- Salt and black pepper to the taste
- 1 teaspoon chili sauce
- 4 endives, trimmed and roughly shredded

Directions:

Grease a pan that fits your air fryer with the oil, add all the ingredients, toss, introduce in the air fryer and cook at 370 degrees F for 20 minutes. Divide everything between plates and serve.

Nutrition: calories 184, fat 2, fiber 2, carbs 3, protein 5

Artichokes Gratin

Prep time: 5 minutes | Cooking time: 15 minutes | Servings: 4

Ingredients:

- 2 tablespoon olive oil
- 12 ounces artichoke hearts
- 4 spring onions, chopped
- Salt and black pepper to the taste
- ½ cup parmesan, grated

Directions:

In a bowl, mix artichoke hearts with the oil, salt, pepper and spring onions and toss. Put the artichokes in your air fryer's basket, sprinkle the parmesan all over and cook at 370 degrees F for 15 minutes. Divide between plates and serve as a side dish.

Nutrition: calories 208, fat 8, fiber 3, carbs 5, protein 8

Artichoke Hearts and Tarragon
Prep time: 5 minutes | Cooking time: 15 minutes | Servings: 4

Ingredients:
- 12 ounces artichoke hearts
- Juice of ½ lemon
- 4 tablespoons butter, melted
- 2 tablespoons tarragon, chopped
- Salt and black pepper to the taste

Directions:
In a bowl, mix all the ingredients, toss, transfer the artichokes to your air fryer's basket and cook at 370 degrees F for 15 minutes. Divide between plates and serve as a side dish.

Nutrition: calories 200, fat 7, fiber 2, carbs 3, protein 7

Coriander Artichokes
Prep time: 5 minutes | Cooking time: 15 minutes | Servings: 4

Ingredients:
- 12 ounces artichoke hearts
- ½ teaspoon olive oil
- 1 teaspoon coriander, ground
- ½ teaspoon cumin seeds
- Salt and black pepper to the taste
- 1 tablespoon lemon juice

Directions:
In a pan that fits your air fryer, mix all the ingredients, toss, introduce the pan in the fryer and cook at 370 degrees F for 15 minutes. Divide the mix between plates and serve as a side dish.

Nutrition: calories 200, fat 7, fiber 2, carbs 5, protein 8

Turmeric Mushroom Mix
Prep time: 5 minutes | Cooking time: 15 minutes | Servings: 4

Ingredients:
- 1 pound brown mushrooms
- 1 teaspoon olive oil
- 4 garlic cloves, minced
- ½ teaspoon turmeric powder
- ¼ teaspoon cinnamon powder
- Salt and black pepper to the taste

Directions:
In a bowl, combine all the ingredients and toss. Put the mushrooms in your air fryer's basket and cook at 370 degrees F for 15 minutes. Divide the mix between plates and serve as a side dish.

Nutrition: calories 208, fat 7, fiber 3, carbs 5, protein 7

Artichokes and Spinach Sauté
Prep time: 5 minutes | Cooking time: 15 minutes | Servings: 4

Ingredients:
- 10 ounces artichoke hearts, halved
- 3 garlic cloves
- 2 cups baby spinach
- ¼ cup veggie stock
- 2 teaspoons lime juice
- Salt and black pepper to the taste

Directions:
In a pan that fits your air fryer, mix all the ingredients, toss, introduce in the fryer and cook at 370 degrees F for 15 minutes. Divide between plates and serve as a side dish.

Nutrition: calories 209, fat 6, fiber 2, carbs 4, protein 8

Ketogenic Air Fryer Snack and Appetizer Recipes

Chicken Cubes
Prep time: 5 minutes | *Cooking time:* 20 minutes | *Servings:* 4

Ingredients:
- 2 teaspoons garlic powder
- 2 eggs
- Salt and black pepper to the taste
- ¾ cup coconut flakes
- Cooking spray
- 1 pound chicken breasts, skinless, boneless and cubed

Directions:
Put the coconut in a bowl and mix the eggs with garlic powder, salt and pepper in a second one. Dredge the chicken cubes in eggs and then in coconut and arrange them all in your air fryer's basket. Grease with cooking spray, cook at 370 degrees F for 20 minutes. Arrange the chicken bites on a platter and serve as an appetizer.

Nutrition: calories 202, fat 12, fiber 2, carbs 4, protein 7

Mexican Chips
Prep time: 5 minutes | *Cooking time:* 5 minutes | *Servings:* 8

Ingredients:
- 2 cups mozzarella, shredded
- ¾ cup almond flour
- 2 teaspoons psyllium husk powder
- ¼ teaspoon sweet paprika

Directions:
Put the mozzarella in a bowl, melt it in the microwave for 2 minutes, add all the other ingredients quickly and stir really until you obtain a dough. Divide the dough into 2 balls, roll them on 2 baking sheets and cut into triangles. Arrange the tortillas in your air fryer's basket and bake at 370 degrees F for 5 minutes. Transfer to bowls and serve as a snack.

Nutrition: calories 170, fat 2, fiber 3, carbs 4, protein 6

Cheese Chips
Prep time: 2 minutes | Cooking time: 5 minutes | Servings: 4

Ingredients:
- 8 ounces cheddar cheese, shredded
- 1 teaspoon sweet paprika

Directions:
Divide the cheese in small heaps in a pan that fits the air fryer, sprinkle the paprika on top, introduce the pan in the machine and cook at 400 degrees F for 5 minutes. Cool the chips down and serve them.

Nutrition: calories 150, fat 4, fiber 3, carbs 4, protein 6

Zucchini and Olives Cakes
Prep time: 5 minutes | Cooking time: 12 minutes | Servings: 6

Ingredients:
- Cooking spray
- ½ cup parsley, chopped
- 1 egg
- ½ cup almond flour
- Salt and black pepper to the taste
- 3 spring onions, chopped
- ½ cup kalamata olives, pitted and minced
- 3 zucchinis, grated

Directions:
In a bowl, mix all the ingredients except the cooking spray, stir well and shape medium cakes out of this mixture. Place the cakes in your air fryer's basket, grease them with cooking spray and cook at 380 degrees F for 6 minutes on each side. Serve them as an appetizer.

Nutrition: calories 165, fat 5, fiber 2, carbs 3, protein 7

Rosemary Mushroom Balls
Prep time: 5 minutes | Cooking time: 12 minutes | Servings: 6

Ingredients:

- Salt and black pepper to the taste
- 1 and ¼ cups coconut flour
- 2 garlic clove, minced
- 2 tablespoons basil, minced
- ½ pound mushrooms, minced
- 1 egg, whisked

Directions:

In a bowl, mix all the ingredients except the cooking spray, stir well and shape medium balls out of this mix. Arrange the balls in your air fryer's basket, grease them with cooking spray and bake at 350 degrees F for 6 minutes on each side. Serve as an appetizer.

Nutrition: calories 151, fat 2, fiber 1, carbs 3, protein 6

Zucchini Chips
Prep time: 5 minutes | Cooking time: 15 minutes | Servings: 6

Ingredients:

- 3 zucchinis, thinly sliced
- Salt and black pepper to the taste
- 2 eggs, whisked
- 1 cup almond flour

Directions:

In a bowl, mix the eggs with salt and pepper. Put the flour in a second bowl. Dredge the zucchinis in flour and then in eggs. Arrange the chips in your air fryer's basket, cook at 350 degrees F for 15 minutes and serve as a snack.

Nutrition: calories 120, fat 4, fiber 2, carbs 3, protein 5

Avocado Wraps
Prep time: 5 minutes | Cooking time: 15 minutes | Servings: 4

Ingredients:
- 2 avocados, peeled, pitted and cut into 12 wedges
- 12 bacon strips
- 1 tablespoon ghee, melted

Directions:
Wrap each avocado wedge in a bacon strip, brush them with the ghee, put them in your air fryer's basket and cook at 360 degrees F for 15 minutes. Serve as an appetizer.

Nutrition: calories 161, fat 4, fiber 2, carbs 4, protein 6

Brussels Sprouts Wraps
Prep time: 5 minutes | Cooking time: 20 minutes | Servings: 12

Ingredients:
- 12 bacon strips
- 12 Brussels sprouts
- A drizzle of olive oil

Directions:
Wrap each Brussels sprouts in a bacon strip, brush them with some oil, put them in your air fryer's basket and cook at 350 degrees F for 20 minutes. Serve as an appetizer.

Nutrition: calories 140, fat 5, fiber 2, carbs 4, protein 4

Bacon Snack
Prep time: 5 minutes | Cooking time: 10 minutes | Servings: 4

Ingredients:
- 4 bacon slices, halved
- 1 cup dark chocolate, melted
- A pinch of pink salt

Directions:
Dip each bacon slice in some chocolate, sprinkle pink salt over them, put them in your air fryer's basket and cook at 350 degrees F for 10 minutes. Serve as a snack.

Nutrition: calories 151, fat 4, fiber 2, carbs 4, protein 8

Pickled Snack

Prep time: 5 minutes | Cooking time: 20 minutes | Servings: 4

Ingredients:

- 4 dill pickle spears, sliced in half and quartered
- 8 bacon slices, halved
- 1 cup avocado mayonnaise

Directions:

Wrap each pickle spear in a bacon slice, put them in your air fryer's basket and cook at 400 degrees F for 20 minutes. Serve as a snack with the mayonnaise.

Nutrition: calories 100, fat 4, fiber 2, carbs 3, protein 4

Avocado Balls

Prep time: 5 minutes | Cooking time: 5 minutes | Servings: 4

Ingredients:

- 1 avocado, peeled, pitted and mashed
- ¼ cup ghee, melted
- 2 garlic cloves, minced
- 2 spring onions, minced
- 1 chili pepper, chopped
- 1 tablespoon lime juice
- 2 tablespoons cilantro
- A pinch of salt and black pepper
- 4 bacon slices, cooked and crumbled
- Cooking spray

Directions:

In a bowl, mix all the ingredients except the cooking spray, stir well and shape medium balls out of this mix. Place them in your air fryer's basket, grease with cooking spray and cook at 370 degrees F for 5 minutes. Serve as a snack.

Nutrition: calories 160, fat 6, fiber 3, carbs 4, protein 6

Shrimp Balls
Prep time: 5 minutes | Cooking time: 15 minutes | Servings: 4

Ingredients:
- 1 pound shrimp, peeled, deveined and minced
- 1 egg, whisked
- 3 tablespoons coconut, shredded
- ½ cup coconut flour
- 1 tablespoon avocado oil
- 1 tablespoon cilantro, chopped

Directions:
In a bowl, mix all the ingredients, stir well and shape medium balls out of this mix. Place the balls in your lined air fryer's basket, cook at 350 degrees F for 15 minutes and serve as an appetizer.

Nutrition: calories 184, fat 5, fiber 2, carbs 4, protein 7

Cilantro Dip
Prep time: 5 minutes | Cooking time: 8 minutes| Servings: 6

Ingredients:
- ½ cup cashews, soaked in water for 4 hours and drained
- 3 tablespoons cilantro, chopped
- 2 garlic cloves, minced
- 1 teaspoon lime juice
- A pinch of salt and black pepper
- 2 tablespoons coconut milk

Directions:
In a blender, combine all the ingredients, pulse well and transfer to a ramekin. Put the ramekin in your air fryer's basket and cook at 350 degrees F for 8 minutes. Serve as a party dip.

Nutrition: calories 144, fat 2, fiber 1, carbs 3, protein 4

Smoked Salmon Bites
Prep time: 5 minutes | Cooking time: 10 minutes | Servings: 12

Ingredients:
- 2 avocados, peeled, pitted and mashed
- 4 ounces smoked salmon, skinless, boneless and chopped
- 2 tablespoons coconut cream
- 1 teaspoon avocado oil
- 1 teaspoon dill, chopped
- A pinch of salt and black pepper

Directions:
In a bowl, mix all the ingredients, stir well and shape medium balls out of this mix. Place them in your air fryer's basket and cook at 350 degrees F for 10 minutes. Serve as an appetizer.

Nutrition: calories 100, fat 2, fiber 1, carbs 2, protein 2

Parsley Meatballs
Prep time: 5 minutes | Cooking time: 20 minutes | Servings: 6

Ingredients:
- 1 pound beef meat, ground
- 1 teaspoon onion powder
- 1 teaspoon garlic powder
- A pinch of salt and black pepper
- 2 tablespoons parsley, chopped
- Cooking spray

Directions:
In a bowl, mix all the ingredients except the cooking spray, stir well and shape medium meatballs out of this mix. Pace them in your lined air fryer's basket, grease with cooking spray and cook at 360 degrees F for 20 minutes. Serve as an appetizer.

Nutrition: calories 180, fat 5, fiber 2, carbs 5, protein 7

Chicken Party Meatballs

Prep time: 5 minutes | Cooking time: 20 minutes | Servings: 12

Ingredients:

- 2 pound chicken breast, skinless, boneless and ground
- A pinch of salt and black pepper
- 2 garlic cloves, minced
- 2 spring onions, chopped
- 2 tablespoons ghee, melted
- 6 tablespoons hot sauce
- ¾ cup almond meal
- Cooking spray

Directions:

In a bowl, mix all the ingredients except the cooking spray, stir well and shape medium meatballs out of this mix. Arrange the meatballs in your air fryer's basket, grease them with cooking spray and cook at 360 degrees F for 20 minutes. Serve as an appetizer.

Nutrition: calories 257, fat 14, fiber 1, carbs 3, protein 17

Chili Meatballs

Prep time: 5 minutes | Cooking time: 20 minutes | Servings: 12

Ingredients:

- 1 pound pork meat, ground
- 3 spring onions, minced
- 3 tablespoons cilantro, chopped
- 1 tablespoon ginger, grated
- 2 garlic cloves, minced
- 1 chili pepper, minced
- A pinch of salt and black pepper
- 1 and ½ tablespoons coconut aminos
- Cooking spray

Directions:

In a bowl, mix all the ingredients except the cooking spray, stir really well and shape medium meatballs out of this mix. Arrange them in your air fryer's basket, grease with cooking spray and cook at 380 degrees F for 20 minutes. Serve as an appetizer.

Nutrition: calories 200, fat 12, fiber 2, carbs 3, protein 14

Asparagus Wraps
Prep time: 5 minutes | Cooking time: 15 minutes | Servings: 8

Ingredients:

- 16 asparagus spears, trimmed
- 16 bacon strips
- 2 tablespoons olive oil
- 1 tablespoon lemon juice
- 1 teaspoon thyme, chopped
- 1 teaspoon oregano, chopped
- A pinch of salt and black pepper

Directions:

In a bowl, mix the oil with lemon juice, the herbs, salt and pepper and whisk well. Brush the asparagus spears with this mix and wrap each in a bacon strip. Arrange the asparagus wraps in your air fryer's basket and cook at 390 degrees F for 15 minutes. Serve as an appetizer.

Nutrition: calories 173, fat 4, fiber 2, carbs 3, protein 6

Radish Chips
Prep time: 5 minutes | Cooking time: 15 minutes | Servings: 4

Ingredients:

- 16 ounces radishes, thinly sliced
- A pinch of salt and black pepper
- 2 tablespoons coconut oil, melted

Directions:

In a bowl, mix the radish slices with salt, pepper and the oil, toss well, place them in your air fryer's basket and cook at 400 degrees F for 15 minutes, flipping them halfway. Serve as a snack.

Nutrition: calories 174, fat 5, fiber 1, carbs 3, protein 6

Olives Dip
Prep time: 5 minutes | Cooking time: 5 minutes | Servings: 6

Ingredients:
- 1 cup black olives, pitted and chopped
- ¼ cup capers
- ½ cup olive oil
- 3 tablespoons lemon juice
- 2 garlic cloves, minced
- 2 teaspoon apple cider vinegar
- 1 cup parsley leaves
- 1 cup basil leaves
- A pinch of salt and black pepper

Directions:
In a blender, combine all the ingredients, pulse well and transfer to a ramekin. Place the ramekin in your air fryer's basket and cook at 350 degrees F for 5 minutes. Serve as a snack.

Nutrition: calories 120, fat 5, fiber 2, carbs 3, protein 7

Warm Tomato Salsa
Prep time: 5 minutes | Cooking time: 8 minutes | Servings: 4

Ingredients:
- 4 tomatoes, cubed
- 3 chili peppers, minced
- 2 spring onions, chopped
- 1 garlic clove, minced
- 2 tablespoons lime juice
- 2 teaspoons cilantro, chopped
- 2 teaspoons parsley, chopped
- Cooking spray

Directions:
Grease a pan that fits your air fryer with the cooking spray, and mix all the ingredients inside. Introduce the pan in the machine and cook at 360 degrees F for 8 minutes. Divide into bowls and serve as an appetizer.

Nutrition: calories 148, fat 1, fiber 2, carbs 3, protein 5

Salmon Spread
Prep time: 5 *minutes* | *Cooking time:* 6 *minutes* | *Servings:* 4

Ingredients:

- 8 ounces cream cheese, soft
- 2 tablespoons lemon juice
- ½ cup coconut cream
- 4 ounces smoked salmon, skinless, boneless and minced
- A pinch of salt and black pepper
- 1 tablespoon chives, chopped

Directions:

In a bowl, mix all the ingredients and whisk them really well. Transfer the mix to a ramekin, place it in your air fryer's basket and cook at 360 degrees F for 6 minutes. Serve as a party spread.

Nutrition: calories 180, fat 7, fiber 1, carbs 5, protein 7

Party Pork Skewers
Prep time: 10 *minutes* | *Cooking time:* 20 *minutes* | *Servings:* 4

Ingredients:

- ½ pound pork shoulder, cubed
- ¼ teaspoon sweet paprika
- 1 tablespoon coconut oil, melted
- ¼ teaspoon cumin, ground
- ¼ cup olive oil
- ¼ cup green bell peppers, chopped
- 1 and ½ tablespoons lemon juice
- 1 tablespoon cilantro, chopped
- 2 tablespoons parsley, chopped
- 2 garlic cloves, minced
- A pinch of salt and black pepper

Directions:

In a blender, combine the olive oil with bell peppers, lemon juice, cilantro, parsley, garlic, salt and pepper and pulse well. Thread the meat onto the skewers, sprinkle cumin and paprika all over and rub with the coconut oil. In a bowl mix the pork skewers with the herbed mix and rub well. Place the skewers in your air fryer's basket, cook at 370 degrees F for 10 minutes on each side and serve as an appetizer.

Nutrition: calories 249, fat 16, fiber 2, carbs 3, protein 17

Spinach Rolls
Prep time: 6 minutes | Cooking time: 20 minutes | Servings: 6

Ingredients:

- 3 cups mozzarella, shredded
- 4 tablespoons coconut flour
- ½ cup almond flour
- 2 eggs, whisked
- A pinch of salt and black pepper
- 6 ounces spinach, chopped
- ¼ cup parmesan, grated
- 4 ounces cream cheese, soft
- 2 tablespoons ghee, melted

Directions:

In a bowl, mix the mozzarella with coconut and almond flour, eggs, salt and pepper, stir well until you obtain a dough and roll it well on a parchment paper. Cut into triangles and leave them aside for now. In a bowl, mix the spinach with parmesan, cream cheese, salt and pepper and stir really well. Divide this into the center of each dough triangle, roll and seal the edges. Brush the rolls with the ghee, place them in your air fryer's basket and cook at 360 degrees F for 20 minutes. Serve as an appetizer.

Nutrition: calories 210, fat 8, fiber 1, carbs 3, protein 8

Pork Belly Bites
Prep time: 10 minutes | Cooking time: 25 minutes | Servings: 6

Ingredients:

- 2 pounds pork belly, cut into strips
- 2 tablespoons olive oil
- 2 teaspoons fennel seeds
- A pinch of salt and black pepper
- A pinch of basil, dried

Directions:

In a bowl, mix all the ingredients, toss and put the pork strips in your air fryer's basket and cook at 425 degrees F for 25 minutes. Divide into bowls and serve as a snack.

Nutrition: calories 251, fat 14, fiber 3, carbs 5, protein 18

Tomato Bites
Prep time: 5 minutes | Cooking time: 20 minutes | Servings: 6

Ingredients:

- 6 tomatoes, halved
- 3 teaspoons sugar-free apricot jam
- 2 ounces watercress
- 2 teaspoons oregano, dried
- 1 tablespoon olive oil
- A pinch of salt and black pepper
- 3 ounces cheddar cheese, grated

Directions:

Spread the jam on each tomato half, sprinkle oregano, salt and pepper, and drizzle the oil all over them Introduce them in the fryer's basket, sprinkle the cheese on top and cook at 360 degrees F for 20 minutes. Arrange the tomatoes on a platter, top each half with some watercress and serve as an appetizer.

Nutrition: calories 131, fat 7, fiber 2, carbs 4, protein 7

Green Beans Snack
Prep time: 5 minutes | Cooking time: 12 minutes | Servings: 4

Ingredients:

- 12 ounces green beans, trimmed
- 1 cup parmesan, grated
- 1 egg, whisked
- A pinch of salt and black pepper
- ¼ teaspoon sweet paprika

Directions:

In a bowl, mix the parmesan with salt, pepper and the paprika and stir. Put the egg in a separate bowl, Dredge the green beans in egg and then in the parmesan mix. Arrange the green beans in your air fryer's basket and cook at 380 degrees F for 12 minutes. Serve as a snack.

Nutrition: calories 112, fat 6, fiber 1, carbs 2, protein 9

Shrimp Snack
Prep time: 5 minutes | Cooking time: 10 minutes | Servings: 4

Ingredients:
- 1 pound shrimp, peeled and deveined
- 3 garlic cloves, minced
- ¼ cup olive oil
- Juice of ½ lemon
- A pinch of salt and black pepper
- ¼ teaspoon cayenne pepper

Directions:
In a pan that fits your air fryer, mix all the ingredients, toss, introduce in the fryer and cook at 370 degrees F for 10 minutes. Serve as a snack.

Nutrition: calories 242, fat 14, fiber 2, carbs 3, protein 17

Mushroom Platter
Prep time: 5 minutes | Cooking time: 12 minutes | Servings: 4

Ingredients:
- 2 tablespoons balsamic vinegar
- 2 tablespoons olive oil
- ½ teaspoon basil, dried
- ½ teaspoon tarragon, dried
- ½ teaspoon rosemary, dried
- ½ teaspoon thyme, dried
- A pinch of salt and black pepper
- 12 ounces Portobello mushrooms, sliced

Directions:
In a bowl, mix all the ingredients and toss well. Arrange the mushroom slices in your air fryer's basket and cook at 380 degrees F for 12 minutes. Arrange the mushroom slices on a platter and serve.

Nutrition: calories 147, fat 8, fiber 2, carbs 3, protein 3

Shrimp and Mushrooms Dip
Prep time: 5 minutes | Cooking time: 20 minutes | Servings: 4

Ingredients:
- 1 pound shrimp, peeled, deveined and minced
- 2 tablespoons ghee, melted
- ¼ pound mushrooms, minced
- ½ cup mozzarella, shredded
- 4 garlic cloves, minced
- 1 tablespoon parsley, chopped
- Salt and black pepper to the taste

Directions:
In a bowl, mix all the ingredients, stir well, divide into small ramekins and place them in your air fryer's basket. Cook at 360 degrees F for 20 minutes and serve as a party dip.

Nutrition: calories 271, fat 15, fiber 3, carbs 4, protein 14

Tuna Appetizer
Prep time: 5 minutes | Cooking time: 10 minutes | Servings: 2

Ingredients:
- 1 pound tuna, skinless, boneless and cubed
- 3 scallion stalks, minced
- 1 chili pepper, minced
- 2 tablespoon olive oil
- 1 tablespoon coconut cream
- 1 tablespoon coconut aminos
- 2 tomatoes, cubed
- 1 teaspoon sesame seeds

Directions:
In a pan that fits your air fryer, mix all the ingredients except the sesame seeds, toss, introduce in the fryer and cook at 360 degrees F for 10 minutes. Divide into bowls and serve as an appetizer with sesame seeds sprinkled on top.

Nutrition: calories 231, fat 18, fiber 3, carbs 4, protein 18

Avocado Bites
Prep time: 5 minutes | Cooking time: 8 minutes | Servings: 4

Ingredients:

- 4 avocados, peeled, pitted and cut into wedges
- 1 egg, whisked
- 1 and ½ cups almond meal
- A pinch of salt and black pepper
- Cooking spray

Directions:

Put the egg in a bowl, and the almond meal in another. Season avocado wedges with salt and pepper, coat them in egg and then in meal almond. Arrange the avocado bites in your air fryer's basket, grease them with cooking spray and cook at 400 degrees F for 8 minutes. Serve as a snack right away.

Nutrition: calories 200, fat 12, fiber 3, carbs 5, protein 16

Onion and Bacon Dip
Prep time: 5 minutes | Cooking time: 20 minutes | Servings: 12

Ingredients:

- 2 tablespoons ghee, melted
- 3 cups spring onions, chopped
- A pinch of salt and black pepper
- 2 ounces cheddar cheese, shredded
- 1/3 cup coconut cream
- 6 bacon slices, cooked and crumbled

Directions:

Heat up a pan that fits the fryer with the ghee over medium-high heat, add the onions, stir and sauté for 7 minutes. Add the remaining ingredients, except the bacon and stir well. Sprinkle the bacon on top, introduce the pan in the machine and cook at and 380 degrees F for 13 minutes. Divide into bowls and serve as a party dip.

Nutrition: calories 220, fat 12, fiber 2, carbs 4, protein 15

Crab and Artichoke Dip

Prep time: 5 minutes | *Cooking time: 20 minutes* | *Servings: 4*

Ingredients:

- 8 ounces cream cheese, soft
- 1 tablespoon lemon juice
- 1 cup coconut cream
- 1 tablespoon lemon juice
- 1 bunch green onions, minced
- 14 ounces canned artichoke hearts, drained and chopped
- 12 ounces jumbo crab meat
- A pinch of salt and black pepper
- 1 and ½ cups mozzarella, shredded

Directions:

In a bowl, combine all the ingredients except half of the cheese and whisk them really well. Transfer this to a pan that fits your air fryer, introduce in the machine and cook at 400 degrees F for 15 minutes. Sprinkle the rest of the mozzarella on top and cook for 5 minutes more. Divide the mix into bowls and serve as a party dip.

Nutrition: calories 240, fat 8, fiber 2, carbs 4, protein 14

Chicken Appetizer Salad

Prep time: 5 minutes | *Cooking time: 20 minutes* | *Servings: 2*

Ingredients:

- 1 chicken breast, skinless, boneless and cut into strips
- 2 cups baby spinach
- 1 cup blueberries
- 6 strawberries, chopped
- ½ cup walnuts, chopped
- 3 tablespoons balsamic vinegar
- 1 tablespoon olive oil
- 3 tablespoons feta cheese, crumbled

Directions:

Heat up a pan that fits the air fryer with the oil over medium heat, add the meat and brown it for 5 minutes. Add the rest of the ingredients except the spinach, toss, introduce in the fryer and cook at 370 degrees F for 15 minutes. Add the spinach, toss, cook for another 5 minutes, divide into bowls and serve.

Nutrition: calories 240, fat 14, fiber 2, carbs 3, protein 12

Tomato and Mozzarella Salad
Prep time: 5 minutes | Cooking time: 12 minutes | Servings: 6

Ingredients:
- 1 pound tomatoes, sliced
- 1 tablespoon balsamic vinegar
- 1 tablespoon ginger, grated
- ½ teaspoon coriander, ground
- 1 teaspoon sweet paprika
- 1 teaspoon chili powder
- 1 cup mozzarella, shredded

Directions:
In a pan that fits your air fryer, mix all the ingredients except the mozzarella, toss, introduce the pan in the air fryer and cook at 360 degrees F for 12 minutes. Divide into bowls and serve cold as an appetizer with the mozzarella sprinkled all over.

Nutrition: calories 185, fat 8, fiber 2, carbs 4, protein 8

Zucchini Salsa
Prep time: 5 minutes | Cooking time: 15 minutes | Servings: 6

Ingredients:
- 1 and ½ pounds zucchinis, roughly cubed
- 2 spring onions, chopped
- 2 tomatoes, cubed
- Salt and black pepper to the taste
- 1 tablespoon balsamic vinegar

Directions:
In a pan that fits your air fryer, mix all the ingredients, toss, introduce the pan in the fryer and cook at 360 degrees F for 15 minutes. Divide the salsa into cups and serve cold.

Nutrition: calories 164, fat 6, fiber 2, carbs 3, protein 8

Cucumber Salsa
Prep time: 5 *minutes* | *Cooking time:* 5 *minutes* | *Servings:* 4

Ingredients:
- 1 and ½ pounds cucumbers, sliced
- 2 spring onions, chopped
- 2 tomatoes cubed
- 2 red chili peppers, chopped
- 2 tablespoons ginger, grated
- 1 tablespoon balsamic vinegar
- A drizzle of olive oil

Directions:
In a pan that fits your air fryer, mix all the ingredients, toss, introduce in the fryer and cook at 340 degrees F for 5 minutes. Divide into bowls and serve cold as an appetizer.

Nutrition: calories 150, fat 2, fiber 1, carbs 2, protein 4

Spinach and Onion Dip
Prep time: 5 *minutes* | *Cooking time:* 20 *minutes* | *Servings:* 6

Ingredients:
- 6 tablespoons ghee, melted
- 1 pound spinach, torn
- 4 spring onions, chopped
- 1 cup mozzarella, shredded
- 1 cup coconut cream
- Salt and black pepper to the taste

Directions:
In a pan that fits the air fryer, combine all the ingredients and whisk them really well. Introduce the pan in your air fryer and cook at 370 degrees F for 20 minutes. Divide into bowls and serve.

Nutrition: calories 184, fat 12, fiber 2, carbs 3, protein 9

Garlic Cheese Dip

Prep time: 5 minutes | Cooking time: 10 minutes | Servings: 10

Ingredients:

- 1 pound mozzarella, shredded
- 1 tablespoon thyme, chopped
- 6 garlic cloves, minced
- 3 tablespoons olive oil
- 1 teaspoon rosemary, chopped
- A pinch of salt and black pepper

Directions:

In a pan that fits your air fryer, mix all the ingredients, whisk really well, introduce in the air fryer and cook at 370 degrees F for 10 minutes. Divide into bowls and serve right away.

Nutrition: calories 184, fat 11, fiber 3, carbs 5, protein 7

Artichokes Dip

Prep time: 5 minutes | Cooking time: 25 minutes | Servings: 6

Ingredients:

- 2 teaspoons olive oil
- 2 spring onions, minced
- 20 ounces canned artichoke hearts, drained and chopped
- 2 garlic cloves, minced
- 6 ounces cream cheese, soft
- ½ cup almond milk
- 1 cup mozzarella, shredded
- A pinch of salt and black pepper

Directions:

Grease a baking pan that fits the air fryer with the oil and mix all the ingredients except the mozzarella inside. Sprinkle the cheese all over, introduce the pan in the air fryer and cook at 370 degrees F for 25 minutes. Divide into bowls and serve as a party dip.

Nutrition: calories 231, fat 11, fiber 2, carbs 4, protein 8

Feta Cheese Dip
Prep time: 5 minutes | *Cooking time:* 5 minutes | *Servings:* 6

Ingredients:

- 2 avocados, peeled, pitted and mashed
- ½ cup feta cheese, crumbled
- ¼ cup spring onion, chopped
- ¼ cup parsley, chopped
- 1 tablespoon jalapeno, minced
- 1 garlic clove, minced
- Juice of 1 lime

Directions:

In a ramekin, mix all the ingredients and whisk them well. Introduce in the fryer and cook at 380 degrees F for 5 minutes. Serve as a party dip right away.

Nutrition: calories 200, fat 12, fiber 2, carbs 4, protein 9

Broccoli Dip
Prep time: 10 minutes | *Cooking time:* 15 minutes | *Servings:* 4

Ingredients:

- 1 and ½ cups veggie stock
- 3 cups broccoli florets
- 2 garlic cloves, minced
- Salt and black pepper to the taste
- 1/3 cup coconut milk
- 1 tablespoon balsamic vinegar
- 1 tablespoon olive oil

Directions:

In a pan that fits your air fryer, mix all the ingredients, toss, introduce in the fryer and cook at 390 degrees F for 15 minutes. Divide into bowls and serve.

Nutrition: calories 163, fat 4, fiber 2, carbs 4, protein 5

Tomatoes Dip
Prep time: 5 minutes | Cooking time: 20 minutes | Servings: 6

Ingredients:

- 1 pint grape tomatoes, halved
- A pinch of salt and black pepper
- 1 teaspoon olive oil
- 12 ounces cream cheese, soft
- 8 ounces mozzarella cheese, grated
- ¼ cup parmesan, grated
- 4 garlic cloves, minced
- 2 tablespoons thyme, chopped
- ¼ cup basil, chopped
- ½ tablespoon oregano, chopped

Directions:

Put the tomatoes in your air fryer's basket and cook them at 400 degrees F for 15 minutes. In a blender, combine the fried tomatoes with the rest of the ingredients and pulse well. Transfer this to a ramekin, place it in the air fryer and cook at 400 degrees F for 5-6 minutes more. Serve as a snack.

Nutrition: calories 184, fat 8, fiber 3, carbs 4, protein 8

Fennel Spread
Prep time: 5 minutes | Cooking time: 25 minutes | Servings: 8

Ingredients:

- 3 tablespoons olive oil
- 3 fennel bulbs, trimmed and cut into wedges
- A pinch of salt and black pepper
- 4 garlic cloves, minced
- ¼ cup parmesan, grated

Directions:

Put the fennel in the air fryer's basket and bake at 380 degrees F for 20 minutes. In a blender, combine the roasted fennel with the rest of the ingredients and pulse well. Put the spread in a ramekin, introduce it in the fryer and cook at 380 degrees F for 5 minutes more. Divide into bowls and serve as a dip.

Nutrition: calories 240, fat 11, fiber 3, carbs 4, protein 12

Cheddar Dip

Prep time: 5 minutes | *Cooking time:* 12 minutes | *Servings:* 6

Ingredients:
- 12 ounces coconut cream
- 2 teaspoons hot sauce
- 8 ounces cheddar cheese, grated

Directions:

In ramekin, mix the cream with hot sauce and cheese and whisk. Put the ramekin in the fryer and cook at 390 degrees F for 12 minutes. Whisk, divide into bowls and serve as a dip.

Nutrition: calories 170, fat 9, fiber 2, carbs 4, protein 12

Peppers and Cheese Dip

Prep time: 5 minutes | *Cooking time:* 20 minutes | *Servings:* 6

Ingredients:
- 8 ounces cream cheese, soft
- 4 ounces parmesan, grated
- 4 ounces mozzarella, grated
- 2 roasted red peppers, chopped
- 2 bacon slices, cooked and crumbled

Directions:

In a pan that fits your air fryer, mix all the ingredients and whisk really well. Introduce the pan in the fryer and cook at 400 degrees F for 20 minutes. Divide into bowls and serve cold.

Nutrition: calories 173, fat 8, fiber 2, carbs 4, protein 11

Cheese and Leeks Dip

Prep time: 5 minutes | *Cooking time:* 12 minutes | *Servings:* 6

Ingredients:
- 2 spring onions, minced
- 2 tablespoons butter, melted
- 3 tablespoons coconut milk
- 4 leeks, sliced
- ¼ cup coconut cream
- Salt and white pepper to the taste

Directions:

In a pan that fits your air fryer, mix all the ingredients and whisk them well. Introduce the pan in the fryer and cook at 390 degrees F for 12 minutes. Divide into bowls and serve.

Nutrition: calories 204, fat 12, fiber 2, carbs 4, protein 14

Turkey and Cheese Balls
Prep time: 5 minutes | *Cooking time:* 20 minutes | *Servings:* 8

Ingredients:

- 2 cups mozzarella, grated
- 1 pound turkey breast, skinless, boneless and ground
- ½ cup almond meal
- ½ cup coconut milk
- 3 tablespoons ghee, melted
- 1 tablespoon Italian seasoning
- 1 teaspoon garlic powder
- ½ cup parmesan, grated
- Cooking spray

Directions:

In a bowl, mix all the ingredients except the parmesan and the cooking spray and stir well. Shape medium balls out of this mix, coat each in the parmesan, and arrange them in your air fryer. Grease the balls with cooking spray and cook at 380 degrees F for 20 minutes. Serve as an appetizer.

Nutrition: calories 210, fat 12, fiber 2, carbs 4, protein 14

Crab Balls
Prep time: 5 minutes | *Cooking time:* 20 minutes | *Servings:* 8

Ingredients:

- ½ cup coconut cream
- 2 tablespoons chives, mined
- 1 egg, whisked
- 1 teaspoon mustard
- 1 teaspoon lemon juice
- 16 ounces lump crab meat, chopped
- 2/3 cup almond meal
- A pinch of salt and black pepper
- Cooking spray

Directions:

In a bowl, mix all the ingredients except the cooking spray and stir well. Shape medium balls out of this mix, place them in the fryer and cook at 390 degrees F for 20 minutes. Serve as an appetizer.

Nutrition: calories 141, fat 7, fiber 2, carbs 4, protein 9

Ketogenic Air Fryer Fish and Seafood Recipes

Parmesan Cod
Prep time: 5 minutes | Cooking time: 15 minutes | Servings: 4

Ingredients:

- 4 cod fillets, boneless
- Salt and black pepper to the taste
- 1 cup parmesan
- 4 tablespoons balsamic vinegar
- A drizzle of olive oil
- 3 spring onions, chopped

Directions:

Season fish with salt, pepper, grease with the oil, and coat it in parmesan. Put the fillets in your air fryer's basket and cook at 370 degrees F for 14 minutes. Meanwhile, in a bowl, mix the spring onions with salt, pepper and the vinegar and whisk. Divide the cod between plates, drizzle the spring onions mix all over and serve with a side salad.

Nutrition: calories 220, fat 12, fiber 2, carbs 5, protein 13

Cod and Spring Onions Sauce
Prep time: 5 minutes | Cooking time: 15 minutes | Servings: 2

Ingredients:

- 2 cod fillets, boneless
- Salt and black pepper to the taste
- 1 bunch spring onions, chopped
- 3 tablespoons ghee, melted

Directions:

In a pan that fits the air fryer, combine all the ingredients, toss gently, introduce in the air fryer and cook at 360 degrees F for 15 minutes. Divide the fish and sauce between plates and serve.

Nutrition: calories 240, fat 12, fiber 2, carbs 5, protein 11

Salmon and Sauce
Prep time: 5 minutes | Cooking time: 20 minutes | Servings: 4

Ingredients:

- 4 salmon fillets, boneless
- A pinch of salt and black pepper
- ½ cup heavy cream
- 1 tablespoon chives, chopped
- 1 teaspoon lemon juice
- 1 teaspoon dill, chopped
- 2 garlic cloves, minced
- ¼ cup ghee, melted

Directions:

In a bowl, mix all the ingredients except the salmon and whisk well. Arrange the salmon in a pan that fits the air fryer, drizzle the sauce all over, introduce the pan in the machine and cook at 360 degrees F for 20 minutes. Divide everything between plates and serve.

Nutrition: calories 220, fat 14, fiber 2, carbs 5, protein 12

Tilapia and Salsa
Prep time: 5 minutes | Cooking time: 15 minutes | Servings: 4

Ingredients:

- 4 tilapia fillets, boneless
- 1 tablespoon olive oil
- A pinch of salt and black pepper
- 12 ounces canned tomatoes, chopped
- 2 tablespoons green onions, chopped
- 2 tablespoons sweet red pepper, chopped
- 1 tablespoon balsamic vinegar

Directions:

Arrange the tilapia in a baking sheet that fits the air fryer and season with salt and pepper. In a bowl, combine all the other ingredients, toss and spread over the fish. Introduce the pan in the fryer and cook at 350 degrees F for 15 minutes. Divide the mix between plates and serve.

Nutrition: calories 221, fat 12, fiber 2, carbs 5, protein 14

Catfish Fillet and Avocado
Prep time: 5 minutes | Cooking time: 15 minutes | Servings: 4

Ingredients:

- 2 teaspoons oregano, dried
- 2 teaspoons cumin, ground
- 2 teaspoons sweet paprika
- A pinch of salt and black pepper
- 4 catfish fillets
- 1 avocado, peeled and cubed
- ½ cup spring onions, chopped
- 2 tablespoons cilantro, chopped
- 2 teaspoons olive oil
- 2 tablespoons lemon juice

Directions:

In a bowl, mix all the ingredients except the fish and toss. Arrange this in a baking pan that fits the air fryer, top with the fish, introduce the pan in the machine and cook at 360 degrees F for 15 minutes, flipping the fish halfway. Divide between plates and serve.

Nutrition: calories 280, fat 14, fiber 3, carbs 5, protein 14

Tilapia and Capers
Prep time: 5 minutes | Cooking time: 20 minutes | Servings: 4

Ingredients:

- 4 tilapia fillets, boneless
- 3 tablespoons ghee, melted
- A pinch of salt and black pepper
- 2 tablespoons capers
- 1 teaspoon garlic powder
- ½ teaspoon smoked paprika
- ½ teaspoon oregano, dried
- 2 tablespoons lemon juice

Directions:

In a bowl, mix all the ingredients except the fish and toss. Arrange the fish in a pan that fits the air fryer, pour the capers mix all over, put the pan in the air fryer and cook 360 degrees F for 20 minutes, shaking halfway. Divide between plates and serve hot.

Nutrition: calories 224, fat 10, fiber 0, carbs 2, protein 18

Glazed Cod Fillets

Prep time: 5 minutes | *Cooking time:* 14 minutes | *Servings:* 4

Ingredients:

- 1/3 cup stevia
- 2 tablespoons coconut aminos
- 4 cod fillets, boneless
- A pinch of salt and black pepper

Directions:

In a pan that fits the air fryer, combine all the ingredients and toss gently. Introduce the pan in the fryer and cook at 350 degrees F for 14 minutes, flipping the fish halfway. Divide everything between plates and serve.

Nutrition: calories 267, fat 18, fiber 2, carbs 5, protein 20

Garlic Tilapia

Prep time: 5 minutes | *Cooking time:* 20 minutes | *Servings:* 4

Ingredients:

- 4 tilapia fillets, boneless
- Salt and black pepper to the taste
- 2 garlic cloves, minced
- 1 teaspoon fennel seeds
- ½ teaspoon red pepper flakes, crushed
- 1 bunch kale, chopped
- 3 tablespoons olive oil

Directions:

In a pan that fits the fryer, combine all the ingredients, put the pan in the fryer and cook at 360 degrees F for 20 minutes. Divide everything between plates and serve.

Nutrition: calories 240, fat 12, fiber 2, carbs 4, protein 12

Paprika Cod
Prep time: 5 minutes | *Cooking time: 14 minutes* | *Servings: 4*

Ingredients:
- 4 cod fillets, boneless
- 1 tablespoon olive oil
- Salt and black pepper to the taste
- 2 teaspoons sweet paprika
- Juice of 1 lime

Directions:
In a bowl, mix all the ingredients, transfer the fish to your air fryer's basket and cook 350 degrees F for 7 minutes on each side. Divide the fish between plates and serve with a side salad.

Nutrition: calories 240, fat 14, fiber 2, carbs 4, protein 16

Salmon Pan
Prep time: 5 minutes | *Cooking time: 12 minutes* | *Servings: 4*

Ingredients:
- 2 tablespoons lime juice
- 1 pound salmon fillets, boneless, skinless and cubed
- 1 tablespoon ginger, grated
- 4 teaspoons olive oil
- 1 tablespoon coconut aminos
- 1 tablespoon sesame seeds, toasted
- 1 tablespoon chives, chopped

Directions:
In a pan that fits the air fryer, combine all the ingredients, toss, introduce in the fryer and cook at 360 degrees F for 12 minutes. Divide into bowls and serve.

Nutrition: calories 206, fat 8, fiber 1, carbs 4, protein 13

Shrimp and Chives
Prep time: 5 minutes | Cooking time: 12 minutes | Servings: 4

Ingredients:
- 1 tablespoon ghee, melted
- 1 pound shrimp, peeled and deveined
- ¼ cup coconut cream
- A pinch of red pepper flakes
- A pinch of salt and black pepper
- 1 tablespoon parsley, chopped
- 1 tablespoon chives, chopped

Directions:
In a pan that fits the fryer, combine all the ingredients except the parsley, put the pan in the fryer and cook at 360 degrees F for 12 minutes. Divide the mix into bowls, sprinkle the parsley on top and serve.

Nutrition: calories 195, fat 11, fiber 2, carbs 4, protein 11

Crispy Salmon Fillets
Prep time: 5 minutes | Cooking time: 15 minutes | Servings: 4

Ingredients:
- 4 salmon fillets, skinless
- 1 teaspoon mustard
- A pinch of salt and black pepper
- ½ cup coconut flakes
- 1 tablespoon parmesan, grated
- Cooking spray

Directions:
In a bowl, mix the parmesan with the other ingredients except the fish and cooking spray and stir well. Coat the fish in this mix, grease it with cooking spray and arrange in the air fryer's basket. Cook at 400 degrees F for 15 minutes, divide between plates and serve with a side salad.

Nutrition: calories 240, fat 13, fiber 3, carbs 6, protein 15

Salmon and Coconut Sauce
Prep time: 5 minutes | Cooking time: 20 minutes | Servings: 4

Ingredients:

- 4 salmon fillets, boneless
- ¼ cup coconut cream
- 1 teaspoon lime zest, grated
- 1/3 cup heavy cream
- ¼ cup lime juice
- ½ cup coconut, shredded
- A pinch of salt and black pepper

Directions:

In a bowl, mix all the ingredients except the salmon and whisk. Arrange the fish in a pan that fits your air fryer, drizzle the coconut sauce all over, put the pan in the machine and cook at 360 degrees F for 20 minutes. Divide between plates and serve.

Nutrition: calories 227, fat 12, fiber 2, carbs 4, protein 9

Mustard Crusted Cod
Prep time: 10 minutes | Cooking time: 14 minutes | Servings: 4

Ingredients:

- 1 cup parmesan, grated
- 4 cod fillets, boneless
- Salt and black pepper to the taste
- 1 tablespoon mustard

Directions:

In a bowl, mix the parmesan with salt, pepper and the mustard and stir. Spread this over the cod, arrange the fish in the air fryer's basket and cook at 370 degrees F for 7 minutes on each side. Divide between plates and serve with a side salad.

Nutrition: calories 270, fat 14, fiber 3, carbs 5, protein 12

Salmon and Shallot Sauce
*Prep time: 5 minutes | **Cooking time:** 15 minutes | Servings: 4*

Ingredients:
- 3 tablespoons parsley, chopped
- 4 salmon fillets, boneless
- ¼ cup ghee, melted
- 2 garlic cloves, minced
- 4 shallots, chopped
- Salt and black pepper to the taste

Directions:
Heat up a pan that fits the air fryer with the ghee over medium-high heat, add the garlic, shallots, salt, pepper and the parsley, stir and cook for 5 minutes. Add the salmon fillets, toss gently, introduce the pan in the air fryer and cook at 380 degrees F for 15 minutes. Divide between plates and serve.

Nutrition: calories 270, fat 12, fiber 2, carbs 4, protein 17

Cod and Endives
*Prep time: 5 minutes | **Cooking time:** 20 minutes | Servings: 4*

Ingredients:
- 2 endives, shredded
- 2 tablespoons olive oil
- Salt and back pepper to the taste
- 4 salmon fillets, boneless
- ½ teaspoon sweet paprika

Directions:
In a pan that fits the air fryer, combine the fish with the rest of the ingredients, toss, introduce in the fryer and cook at 350 degrees F for 20 minutes, flipping the fish halfway. Divide between plates and serve right away.

Nutrition: calories 243, fat 13, fiber 3, carbs 6, protein 14

Tuna Kabobs
Prep time: 5 *minutes* | *Cooking time:* 12 *minutes* | *Servings:* 4

Ingredients:
- 1 pound tuna steaks, boneless and cubed
- 1 chili pepper, minced
- 4 green onions, chopped
- 2 tablespoons lime juice
- A drizzle of olive oil
- Salt and black pepper to the taste

Directions:

In a bowl mix all the ingredients and toss them. Thread the tuna cubes on skewers, arrange them in your air fryer's basket and cook at 370 degrees F for 12 minutes. Divide between plates and serve with a side salad.

Nutrition: calories 226, fat 12, fiber 2, carbs 4, protein 15

Cod and Tomatoes
Prep time: 5 *minutes* | *Cooking time:* 15 *minutes* | *Servings:* 4

Ingredients:
- 1 cup cherry tomatoes, halved
- Salt and black pepper to the taste
- 2 tablespoons olive oil
- 4 cod fillets, skinless and boneless
- 2 tablespoons cilantro, chopped

Directions:

In a baking dish that fits your air fryer, mix all the ingredients, toss gently, introduce in your air fryer and cook at 370 degrees F for 15 minutes. Divide everything between plates and serve right away.

Nutrition: calories 248, fat 11, fiber 2, carbs 5, protein 11

Tilapia and Tomato Mix
Prep time: 5 minutes | *Cooking time: 20 minutes* | *Servings: 4*

Ingredients:

- 4 tilapia fillets, boneless and halved
- Salt and black pepper to the taste
- 1 cup roasted peppers, chopped
- ¼ cup tomato paste
- 1 cup tomatoes, cubed
- 1 tablespoon lemon juice
- 2 tablespoons olive oil
- 1 teaspoon garlic powder
- 1 teaspoon oregano, dried

Directions:

In a baking dish that fits your air fryer, mix the fish with all the other ingredients, toss, introduce in your air fryer and cook at 380 degrees F for 20 minutes. Divide into bowls and serve.

Nutrition: calories 250, fat 9, fiber 2, carbs 5, protein 14

Shrimp and Lemon Vinaigrette
Prep time: 5 minutes | *Cooking time: 12 minutes* | *Servings: 4*

Ingredients:

- 1 and ½ pounds shrimp, peeled and deveined
- Zest of ½ lemon, grated
- Juice of ½ lemon
- A pinch of salt and black pepper
- 2 tablespoons mustard
- 2 tablespoons olive oil
- 2 tablespoons parsley, chopped

Directions:

In a bowl, mix all the ingredients and toss well. Put the shrimp in your air fryer's basket and reserve the lemon vinaigrette. Cook at 350 degrees F for 12 minutes, flipping the shrimp halfway, divide between plates and serve with reserved vinaigrette drizzled on top.

Nutrition: calories 202, fat 8, fiber 2, carbs 5, protein 14

Garlic Shrimp
Prep time: 5 minutes | Cooking time: 12 minutes | Servings: 4

Ingredients:

- 1 pound shrimp, peeled and deveined
- 1 teaspoon cumin, ground
- 2 tablespoons parsley, chopped
- 2 tablespoons olive oil
- A pinch of salt and black pepper
- 4 garlic cloves, minced
- 1 tablespoon lime juice

Directions:

In a pan that fits your air fryer, mix all the ingredients, toss, put the pan in your air fryer and cook at 370 degrees F and cook for 12 minutes, shaking the fryer halfway. Divide into bowls and serve.

Nutrition: calories 220, fat 11, fiber 2, carbs 5, protein 12

Shrimp and Green Beans
Prep time: 5 minutes | Cooking time: 15 minutes | Servings: 4

Ingredients:

- 1 pound shrimp, peeled and deveined
- A pinch of salt and black pepper
- ½ pound green beans, trimmed and halved
- Juice of 1 lime
- 2 tablespoons cilantro, chopped
- ¼ cup ghee, melted

Directions:

In a pan that fits your air fryer, mix all the ingredients, toss, introduce in the fryer and cook at 360 degrees F for 15 minutes shaking the fryer halfway. Divide into bowls and serve.

Nutrition: calories 222, fat 8, fiber 3, carbs 5, protein 10

Sesame Shrimp
Prep time: 3 minutes | Cooking time: 12 minutes | Servings: 4

Ingredients:
- 1 pound shrimp, peeled and deveined
- A pinch of salt and black pepper
- 1 tablespoon sesame seeds, toasted
- ½ teaspoon Italian seasoning
- 1 tablespoon olive oil

Directions:
In a bowl, mix the shrimp with the rest of the ingredients and toss well. Put the shrimp in the air fryer's basket, cook at 370 degrees F for 12 minutes, divide into bowls and serve,

Nutrition: calories 199, fat 11, fiber 2, carbs 4, protein 11

Hot Basil Cod
Prep time: 5 minutes | Cooking time: 15 minutes | Servings: 4

Ingredients:
- 4 cod fillets, boneless
- 1 teaspoon red pepper flakes
- ½ teaspoon hot paprika
- 2 tablespoon olive oil
- 1 teaspoon basil, dried
- Salt and black pepper to the taste

Directions:
In a bowl, mix the cod with all the other ingredients and toss. Put the fish in your air fryer's basket and cook at 380 degrees F for 15 minutes. Divide the cod between plates and serve.

Nutrition: calories 194, fat 7, fiber 2, carbs 4, protein 12

Rosemary Shrimp and Tomatoes
Prep time: 5 minutes | *Cooking time: 12 minutes* | *Servings: 4*

Ingredients:

- 1 pound shrimp, peeled and deveined
- 1 cup cherry tomatoes, halved
- 4 garlic cloves, minced
- Salt and black pepper to the taste
- 1 tablespoon rosemary, chopped
- 2 tablespoons ghee, melted

Directions:

In a pan that fits the air fryer, mix all the ingredients, toss, put the pan in the fryer and cook at 380 degrees F for 12 minutes. Divide into bowls and serve hot.

Nutrition: calories 220, fat 14, fiber 2, carbs 6, protein 15

Shrimp and Pesto
Prep time: 5 minutes | *Cooking time: 12 minutes* | *Servings: 4*

Ingredients:

- ½ cup parsley leaves
- ½ cup basil leaves
- 2 tablespoons lemon juice
- 1/3 cup pine nuts
- ¼ cup parmesan, grated
- A pinch of salt and black pepper
- ½ cup olive oil
- 1 and ½ pounds shrimp, peeled and deveined
- ¼ teaspoon lemon zest, grated

Directions:

In a blender, combine all the ingredients except the shrimp and pulse well. In a bowl, mix the shrimp with the pesto and toss. Put the shrimp in your air fryer's basket and cook at 360 degrees F for 12 minutes, flipping the shrimp halfway. Divide the shrimp into bowls and serve.

Nutrition: calories 240, fat 10, fiber 1, carbs 4, protein 12

Salmon and Green Olives
Prep time: 5 minutes | Cooking time: 15 minutes | Servings: 4

Ingredients:
- 1 tablespoon lemon zest, grated
- 1/3 cup olive oil
- 4 salmon fillets, boneless
- 1 cup green olives, pitted and sliced
- Juice of 2 limes
- Salt and black pepper to the taste

Directions:
In a baking dish that fits your air fryer, mix all the ingredients, toss, put the pan in the fryer and cook at 370 degrees F for 15 minutes. Divide everything between plates and serve.

Nutrition: calories 204, fat 12, fiber 3, carbs 5, protein 15

Shrimp and Zucchinis
Prep time: 5 minutes | Cooking time: 15 minutes | Servings: 4

Ingredients:
- 1 pound shrimp, peeled and deveined
- A pinch of salt and black pepper
- 2 zucchinis, cut into medium cubes
- 1 tablespoon lemon juice
- 1 tablespoon olive oil
- 1 tablespoon garlic, minced

Directions:
In a pan that fits the air fryer, combine all the ingredients, toss, put the pan in the machine and cook at 370 degrees F for 15 minutes. Divide between plates and serve right away.

Nutrition: calories 221, fat 9, fiber 2, carbs 15, protein 11

Shrimp and Black Olives
Prep time: 5 minutes | Cooking time: 12 minutes | Servings: 4

Ingredients:
- 1 pound shrimp, peeled and deveined
- 4 garlic clove, minced
- 1 cup black olives, pitted and chopped
- 3 tablespoons parsley
- 1 tablespoon olive oil

Directions:

In a pan that fits the air fryer, combine all the ingredients, toss, put the pan in the machine and cook at 380 degrees F for 12 minutes. Divide between plates and serve.

Nutrition: calories 251, fat 12, fiber 3, carbs 6, protein 15

Salmon and Cauliflower Rice
Prep time: 5 minutes | Cooking time: 25 minutes | Servings: 4

Ingredients:
- 4 salmon fillets, boneless
- Salt and black pepper to the taste
- 1 cup cauliflower, riced
- ½ cup chicken stock
- 1 teaspoon turmeric powder
- 1 tablespoon butter, melted

Directions:

In a pan that fits your air fryer, mix the cauliflower rice with the other ingredients except the salmon and toss. Arrange the salmon fillets over the cauliflower rice, put the pan in the fryer and cook at 360 degrees F for 25 minutes, flipping the fish after 15 minutes. Divide everything between plates and serve.

Nutrition: calories 241, fat 12, fiber 2, carbs 6, protein 12

Trout and Mint Mix

Prep time: 5 minutes | Cooking time: 16 minutes | Servings: 4

Ingredients:

- 4 rainbow trout
- 1 cup olive oil+ 3 tablespoons
- Juice of 1 lemon
- A pinch of salt and black pepper
- 1 cup parsley, chopped
- 3 garlic cloves, minced
- ½ cup mint, chopped
- Zest of 1 lemon
- 1/3 pine nuts
- 1 avocado, peeled, pitted and roughly chopped

Directions:

Pat dry the trout, season with salt and pepper and rub with 3 tablespoons oil. Put the fish in your air fryer's basket and cook for 8 minutes on each side. Divide the fish between plates and drizzle half of the lemon juice all over. In a blender, combine the rest of the oil with the remaining lemon juice, parsley, garlic, mint, lemon zest, pine nuts and the avocado and pulse well. Spread this over the trout and serve.

Nutrition: calories 240, fat 12, fiber 4, carbs 6, protein 9

Herbed Trout and Asparagus

Prep time: 5 minutes | Cooking time: 20 minutes | Servings: 4

Ingredients:

- 4 trout fillets, boneless and skinless
- 1 tablespoon lemon juice
- 2 tablespoons olive oil
- A pinch of salt and black pepper
- 1 bunch asparagus, trimmed
- 2 tablespoons ghee, melted
- ¼ cup mixed chives and tarragon

Directions:

Mix the asparagus with half of the oil, salt and pepper, put it in your air fryer's basket, cook at 380 degrees F for 6 minutes and divide between plates. In a bowl, mix the trout with salt, pepper, lemon juice, the rest of the oil and the herbes and toss, Put the fillets in your air fryer's basket and cook at 380 degrees F for 7 minutes on each side. Divide the fish next to the asparagus, drizzle the melted ghee all over and serve.

Nutrition: calories 240, fat 12, fiber 4, carbs 6, protein 9

Chives Salmon
Prep time: 5 minutes | Cooking time: 12 minutes | Servings: 4

Ingredients:
- 4 salmon fillets, boneless
- Juice of ½ lemon
- ¼ cup chives, chopped
- 4 cilantro springs, chopped
- 3 tablespoons olive oil
- Salt and black pepper to the taste

Directions:
In a bowl, mix the salmon with all the other ingredients and toss. Put the fillets in your air fryer's basket and cook at 370 degrees F for 12 minutes, flipping the fish halfway. Divide everything between plates and serve with a side salad.

Nutrition: calories 240, fat 12, fiber 5, carbs 6, protein 14

Trout Fillets and Bell Peppers
Prep time: 5 minutes | Cooking time: 16 minutes | Servings: 2

Ingredients:
- 2 trout fillets, boneless
- 2 tomatoes, cubed
- 1 red bell pepper, chopped
- 2 garlic cloves, minced
- 1 tablespoon olive oil
- 1 tablespoon balsamic vinegar
- A pinch of salt and black pepper
- 2 tablespoon almond flakes

Directions:
Arrange the fish in a pan that fits your air fryer, add the rest of the ingredients and toss gently. Cook at 370 degrees F for 16 minutes, divide between plates and serve.

Nutrition: calories 261, fat 14, fiber 5, carbs 6, protein 14

Trout and Almonds
Prep time: 5 minutes | Cooking time: 15 minutes | Servings: 2

Ingredients:

- 2 trout fillets, boneless
- 2 tablespoons almonds, crushed
- Zest of ½ lemon, grated
- 1 tablespoon olive oil
- 1 tablespoon ghee, melted
- A pinch of salt and black pepper
- 1 tablespoon parsley, chopped

Directions:

In a bowl, mix the trout with all the other ingredients except the parsley and toss. Put the fish in your air fryer's basket and cook at 370 degrees F for 15 minutes, flipping the fillets halfway. Divide between plates, sprinkle the parsley on top and serve.

Nutrition: calories 271, fat 13, fiber 4, carbs 6, protein 12

Sea Bass and Fennel
Prep time: 5 minutes | Cooking time: 20 minutes | Servings: 2

Ingredients:

- 2 sea bass, fillets
- 1 fennel bulb, sliced
- Juice of 1 lemon
- ¼ cup black olives, pitted and sliced
- 1 tablespoon olive oil
- A pinch of salt and black pepper
- ¼ cup basil, chopped

Directions:

In a pan that fits the air fryer, combine all the ingredients, introduce the pan in the machine and cook at 380 degrees F for 20 minutes, shaking the fryer halfway. Divide between plates and serve.

Nutrition: calories 254, fat 10, fiber 4, carbs 6, protein 11

Sea Bass and Risotto
Prep time: 5 minutes | *Cooking time:* 25 minutes | *Servings:* 4

Ingredients:

- 4 sea bass fillets, boneless
- A pinch of salt and black pepper
- 1 tablespoon ghee, melted
- 1 garlic clove, minced
- 1 cup cauliflower rice
- ½ cup chicken stock
- 1 tablespoon parmesan, grated
- 1 tablespoon chervil, chopped
- 1 tablespoon parsley, chopped
- 1 tablespoon tarragon, chopped

Directions:

In a pan that fits your air fryer, mix the cauliflower rice with the stock, parmesan, chervil, tarragon and parsley, toss, introduce the pan in the air fryer and cook at 380 degrees F for 12 minutes. In a bowl, mix the fish with salt, pepper, garlic and melted ghee and toss gently. Put the fish over the cauliflower rice, cook at 380 degrees F for 12 minutes more, divide everything between plates and serve.

Nutrition: calories 261, fat 12, fiber 4, carbs 6, protein 11

Fish Fillets and Coconut Sauce
Prep time: 5 minutes | *Cooking time:* 20 minutes | *Servings:* 4

Ingredients:

- 4 sea bass fillets, boneless
- A pinch of salt and black pepper
- 2 spring onions, chopped
- Juice of 1 lime
- 1 garlic clove, minced
- 2 tomatoes, cubed
- 2 cups coconut cream
- ½ cup okra
- A handful coriander, chopped
- 2 red chilies, minced

Directions:

Put the coconut cream in a pan that fits the air fryer, add garlic, spring onions, lime juice, tomatoes, okra, chilies and the coriander, toss, bring to a simmer and cook for 5-6 minutes. Add the fish, toss gently, introduce in the fryer and cook at 380 degrees F for 15 minutes. Divide between plates and serve.

Nutrition: calories 261, fat 12, fiber 5, carbs 6, protein 11

Clams and Cilantro Sauce
Prep time: 5 minutes | Cooking time: 20 minutes | Servings: 4

Ingredients:

- 15 small clams
- 1 tablespoon spring onions, chopped
- Juice of 1 lime
- 10 ounces coconut cream
- 2 tablespoons cilantro, chopped
- 1 teaspoon olive oil

Directions:

Heat up a pan that fits your air fryer with the oil over medium heat, add the spring onions and sauté for 2 minutes. Add lime juice, coconut cream and the cilantro, stir and cook for 2 minutes more. Add the clams, toss, introduce in the fryer and cook at 390 degrees F for 15 minutes. Divide into bowls and serve hot.

Nutrition: calories 231, fat 6, fiber 2, carbs 6, protein 10

Mediterranean Cod Fillets
Prep time: 5 minutes | Cooking time: 15 minutes | Servings: 4

Ingredients:

- 4 cod fillets, boneless
- A pinch of salt and black pepper
- 1 tablespoon thyme, chopped
- ½ teaspoon black peppercorns
- 2 tablespoons olive oil
- 1 fennel, sliced
- 2 garlic cloves, minced
- 1 red bell pepper, chopped
- 2 teaspoons Italian seasoning

Directions:

In a bowl, mix the fennel with bell pepper and the other ingredients except the fish fillets and toss. Put this into a pan that fits the air fryer, add the fish on top, introduce the pan in your air fryer and cook at 380 degrees F for 15 minutes. Divide between plates and serve.

Nutrition: calories 241, fat 12, fiber 4, carbs 7, protein 11

Lemongrass Sea Bass
Prep time: 5 minutes | Cooking time: 15 minutes | Servings: 4

Ingredients:
- 4 sea bass fillets, boneless
- 4 garlic cloves, minced
- Juice of 1 lime
- 1 cup veggie stock
- A pinch of salt and black pepper
- 1 tablespoon black peppercorns, crushed
- 1-inch ginger, grated
- 4 lemongrass, chopped
- 4 small chilies, minced
- 1 bunch coriander, chopped

Directions:
In a blender, combine all the ingredients except the fish and pulse well. Pour the mix in a pan that fits the air fryer, add the fish, toss, introduce in the fryer and cook at 380 degrees F for 15 minutes. Divide between plates and serve.

Nutrition: calories 271, fat 12, fiber 4, carbs 6, protein 12

Italian Shrimp
Prep time: 5 minutes | Cooking time: 10 minutes | Servings: 4

Ingredients:
- 2 pounds shrimp, peeled and deveined
- A drizzle of olive oil
- ¼ cup chicken stock
- 1 tablespoon Italian seasoning
- Salt and black pepper to the taste
- 1 teaspoon red pepper flakes, crushed
- 8 garlic cloves, crushed

Directions:
Grease a pan that fits your air fryer with the oil, add the shrimp and the rest of the ingredients, toss, introduce the pan in the fryer and cook at 390 degrees F for 10 minutes. Divide into bowls and serve.

Nutrition: calories 261, fat 12, fiber 6, carbs 7, protein 12

Simple Shrimp
Prep time: 3 minutes | Cooking time: 10 minutes | Servings: 4

Ingredients:
- 1 pound shrimp, peeled and deveined
- 2 tablespoons olive oil
- 1 tablespoon red onion, chopped
- 1 cup chicken stock

Directions:

In a pan that fits your air fryer, mix the shrimp with the oil, onion and the stock, introduce the pan in the fryer and cook at 380 degrees F for 10 minutes. Divide into bowls and serve.

Nutrition: calories 261, fat 6, fiber 8, carbs 16, protein 6

Fish and Salsa
Prep time: 5 minutes | Cooking time: 15 minutes | Servings: 4

Ingredients:
- 4 sea bass fillets, boneless
- 1 tablespoon olive oil
- 3 tomatoes, roughly chopped
- 2 spring onions, chopped
- ¼ cup chicken stock
- A pinch of salt and black pepper
- 3 garlic cloves, minced
- 1 tablespoon balsamic vinegar

Directions:

In a blender, combine all the ingredients except the fish and pulse well. Put the mix in a pan that fits the air fryer, add the fish, toss gently, introduce the pan in the fryer and cook at 380 degrees F for 15 minutes. Divide between plates and serve.

Nutrition: calories 261, fat 11, fiber 4, carbs 7, protein 11

Simple Flounder Fillets
Prep time: 5 minutes | Cooking time: 20 minutes | Servings: 4

Ingredients:
- 4 flounder fillets, boneless
- A pinch of salt and black pepper
- 1 cup parmesan, grated
- 4 tablespoons butter, melted
- 2 tablespoons olive oil

Directions:
In a bowl, mix the parmesan with salt, pepper, butter and the oil and stir well. Arrange the fish in a pan that fits the air fryer, spread the parmesan mix all over, introduce in the fryer and cook at 400 degrees F for 20 minutes. Divide between plates and serve with a side salad.

Nutrition: calories 251, fat 14, fiber 5, carbs 6, protein 12

Shrimp and Okra
Prep time: 5 minutes | Cooking time: 10 minutes | Servings: 4

Ingredients:
- 1 pound shrimp, peeled and deveined
- 2 tablespoons coconut aminos
- 1 and ½ cups okra
- 3 tablespoons balsamic vinegar
- ½ cup chicken stock
- A pinch of salt and black pepper
- 1 tablespoon parsley, chopped

Directions:
In a pan that fits your air fryer, mix all the ingredients, toss, introduce in the fryer and cook at 380 degrees F for 10 minutes. Divide into bowls and serve.

Nutrition: calories 251, fat 10, fiber 3, carbs 4, protein 8

Lemony Flounder Fillets
Prep time: 5 *minutes* | *Cooking time:* 12 *minutes* | *Servings:* 2

Ingredients:
- 2 flounder fillets, boneless
- 2 garlic cloves, minced
- 2 teaspoons coconut aminos
- 2 tablespoons lemon juice
- A pinch of salt and black pepper
- ½ teaspoon stevia
- 2 tablespoons olive oil

Directions:
In a pan that fits your air fryer, mix all the ingredients, toss, introduce in the fryer and cook at 390 degrees F for 12 minutes. Divide into bowls and serve.

Nutrition: calories 251, fat 13, fiber 3, carbs 5, protein 10

Flounder Fillets and Mushrooms
Prep time: 5 *minutes* | *Cooking time:* 15 *minutes* | *Servings:* 4

Ingredients:
- 4 flounder fillets, boneless
- 2 tablespoons coconut aminos
- A pinch of salt and black pepper
- 1 and ½ teaspoons ginger, grated
- 2 teaspoons olive oil
- 2 green onions, chopped
- 2 cups mushrooms, sliced

Directions:
Heat u a pan that fits your air fryer with the oil over medium-high heat, add the mushrooms and all the other ingredients except the fish, toss and sauté for 5 minutes. Add the fish, toss gently, introduce the pan in the fryer and cook at 390 degrees F for 10 minutes. Divide between plates and serve.

Nutrition: calories 271, fat 12, fiber 4, carbs 6, protein 11

Butter Trout
Prep time: 10 minutes | Cooking time: 12 minutes | Servings: 4

Ingredients:
- 4 trout fillets, boneless
- 4 tablespoons butter, melted
- Salt and black pepper to the taste
- Juice of 1 lime
- 1 tablespoon chives, chopped
- 1 tablespoon parsley, chopped

Directions:
Mix the fish fillets with the melted butter, salt and pepper, rub gently, put the fish in your air fryer's basket and cook at 390 degrees F for 6 minutes on each side. Divide between plates and serve with lime juice drizzled on top and with parsley and chives sprinkled at the end.

Nutrition: calories 221, fat 11, fiber 4, carbs 6, protein 9

Tarragon and Parmesan Trout
Prep time: 5 minutes | Cooking time: 15 minutes | Servings: 4

Ingredients:
- 2 tablespoons olive oil
- 2 garlic cloves, minced
- ½ cup chicken stock
- Salt and black pepper to the taste
- 4 trout fillets, boneless
- ¾ cup parmesan, grated
- ¼ cup tarragon, chopped

Directions:
In a pan that fits your air fryer, mix all the ingredients except the fish and the parmesan and whisk. Add the fish and grease it well with this mix. Sprinkle the parmesan on top, put the pan in the air fryer and cook at 380 degrees F for 15 minutes. Divide everything between plates and serve.

Nutrition: calories 271, fat 12, fiber 4, carbs 6, protein 11

Crab and Tomato Sauce
Prep time: 5 minutes | Cooking time: 20 minutes | Servings: 4

Ingredients:
- 2 tablespoons olive oil
- 1 cup green bell pepper, chopped
- 4 garlic cloves, chopped
- 8 tomatoes, chopped
- ½ teaspoon garlic powder
- 1 teaspoon thyme, dried
- 1 teaspoon sweet paprika
- ¼ cup chicken stock
- 1 and ½ pound crab meat
- A pinch of salt and black pepper
- 1 tablespoon chives, chopped

Directions:
Heat up a pan that fist the air fryer with the oil over medium heat, add bell pepper and the garlic and sauté for 2 minutes. Add the rest of the ingredients except the crab meat, stir, bring to a boil and simmer for 6 minutes more. Add the crab meat, put the pan in the fryer and cook at 380 degrees F for 15 minutes. Divide into bowls and serve.

Nutrition: calories 261, fat 11, fiber 4, carbs 6, protein 10

Baked Black Sea Bass
Prep time: 5 minutes | Cooking time: 20 minutes | Servings: 4

Ingredients:
- 4 black sea bass fillets, boneless
- 1 pound broccoli florets
- 4 tablespoons butter, melted
- ½ teaspoon red pepper flakes, crushed
- 1 teaspoon lemon zest, grated
- A pinch of salt and black pepper

Directions:
In a pan that fits your air fryer, mix the broccoli with the other ingredients except the fish and half of the butter, toss, put the pan in the fryer and cook at 380 degrees F for 8 minutes. Add the fish greased with the rest of the butter, cook at 380 degrees F for 12 minutes more, divide between plates and serve.

Nutrition: calories 251, fat 15, fiber 4, carbs 6, protein 12

Snapper and Spring Onions Mix
Prep time: 5 minutes | Cooking time: 14 minutes | Servings: 4

Ingredients:

- 4 snapper fillets, boneless and skin scored
- 2 tablespoons sweet paprika
- 3 tablespoons olive oil
- A pinch of salt and black pepper
- 6 spring onions, chopped
- Juice of ½ lemon

Directions:

In a bowl, mix the paprika with the rest of the ingredients except the fish and whisk well. Rub the fish with this mix, place the fillets in your air fryer's basket and cook at 390 degrees F for 7 minutes on each side. Divide between plates and serve with a side salad.

Nutrition: calories 241, fat 12, fiber 4, carbs 6, protein 13

Roasted Char Fillets
Prep time: 5 minutes | Cooking time: 18 minutes | Servings: 4

Ingredients:

- 4 char fillets, boneless
- 3 tablespoons olive oil
- 1 fennel bulb, sliced with a mandoline
- A pinch of salt and black pepper
- 5 garlic cloves, minced
- 1 teaspoon caraway seeds
- 2 tablespoons balsamic vinegar
- 1 tablespoon lemon juice
- 1 tablespoon lemon peel, grated
- ½ cup dill, chopped

Directions:

In a pan that fits your air fryer, mix the fish with all the other ingredients, toss, introduce in the air fryer and cook at 390 degrees F for 18 minutes. Divide the fish between plates and serve with a side salad.

Nutrition: calories 251, fat 16, fiber 4, carbs 6, protein 13

Hot Roasted Red Snapper

Prep time: 5 minutes | Cooking time: 15 minutes | Servings: 4

Ingredients:

- 4 red snapper fillets, boneless
- A pinch of salt and black pepper
- 2 garlic cloves, minced
- 2 tablespoons coconut aminos
- 2 tablespoons lime juice
- 1 tablespoon hot chili paste
- 2 tablespoons olive oil

Directions:

In a bowl, mix all the ingredients except the fish and whisk well. Rub the fish with this mix, place it in your air fryer's basket and cook at 380 degrees F for 15 minutes. Serve with a side salad.

Nutrition: calories 220, fat 13, fiber 4, carbs 6, protein 11

Herbed Halibut

Prep time: 5 minutes | Cooking time: 18 minutes | Servings: 4

Ingredients:

- 4 halibut fillets, boneless
- A pinch of salt and black pepper
- 1 shallot, chopped
- 2 garlic cloves, minced
- 1 cup parsley, chopped
- 1 tablespoon chives, chopped
- 1 tablespoon lemon zest, grated
- 1 tablespoon capers, drained and chopped
- 1 tablespoon lemon juice
- 1 tablespoon olive oil
- 1 tablespoon butter, melted

Directions:

Heat up a pan that fits your air fryer with the oil and the butter over medium-high heat, add the shallot and the garlic and sauté for 2 minutes. Add the rest of the ingredients except the fish, toss and sauté for 3 minutes more. Add the fish, sear for 1 minute on each side, toss it gently with the herbed mix, place the pan in the air fryer and cook at 380 degrees F for 12 minutes. Divide everything between plates and serve.

Nutrition: calories 220, fat 12, fiber 2, carbs 6, protein 10

Swordfish Steaks and Tomatoes
Prep time: 5 minutes | Cooking time: 10 minutes | Servings: 2

Ingredients:

- 2 1-inch thick swordfish steaks
- A pinch of salt and black pepper
- 30 ounces canned tomatoes, chopped
- 2 tablespoons capers, drained
- 1 tablespoon red vinegar
- 2 tablespoons oregano, chopped

Directions:

In a pan that fits the air fryer, combine all the ingredients, toss, put the pan in the fryer and cook at 390 degrees F for 10 minutes, flipping the fish halfway. Divide the mix between plates and serve.

Nutrition: calories 280, fat 12, fiber 4, carbs 6, protein 11

Basil Swordfish Fillets
Prep time: 5 minutes | Cooking time: 12 minutes | Servings: 4

Ingredients:

- 4 swordfish fillets, boneless
- 1 tablespoon olive oil
- ¾ teaspoon sweet paprika
- 2 teaspoons basil, dried
- Juice of 1 lemon
- 2 tablespoons butter, melted

Directions:

In a bowl, mix the oil with the other ingredients except the fish fillets and whisk. Brush the fish with this mix, place it in your air fryer's basket and cook for 6 minutes on each side. Divide between plates and serve with a side salad.

Nutrition: calories 216, fat 11, fiber 3, carbs 6, protein 12

Lime Trout and Shallots
Prep time: 5 minutes | Cooking time: 12 minutes | Servings: 4

Ingredients:
- 4 trout fillets, boneless
- Juice of 1 lime
- ½ cup butter, melted
- ½ cup olive oil
- 3 garlic cloves, minced
- 6 shallots, chopped
- A pinch of salt and black pepper

Directions:
In a pan that fits the air fryer, combine the fish with the shallots and the rest of the ingredients, toss gently, put the pan in the machine and cook at 390 degrees F for 12 minutes, flipping the fish halfway. Divide between plates and serve with a side salad.

Nutrition: calories 270, fat 12, fiber 4, carbs 6, protein 12

Black Sea Bass with Rosemary Vinaigrette
Prep time: 5 minutes | Cooking time: 12 minutes | Servings: 4

Ingredients:
- 4 black sea bass fillets, boneless and skin scored
- 2 tablespoons olive oil
- A pinch of salt and black pepper
- 3 tablespoons black olives, pitted and chopped
- 3 garlic cloves, minced
- 1 tablespoon rosemary, chopped
- Juice of 1 lime

Directions:
In a bowl, mix the oil with the olives and the rest of the ingredients except the fish and whisk well. Place the fish in a pan that fits the air fryer, spread the rosemary vinaigrette all over, put the pan in the machine and cook at 380 degrees F for 12 minutes, flipping the fish halfway. Divide between plates and serve.

Nutrition: calories 220, fat 12, fiber 4, carbs 6, protein 10

Trout and Zucchinis
Prep time: 5 minutes | Cooking time: 15 minutes | Servings: 4

Ingredients:

- 3 zucchinis, cut in medium chunks
- 4 trout fillets, boneless
- 2 tablespoons olive oil
- ¼ cup tomato sauce
- Salt and black pepper to the taste
- 1 garlic clove, minced
- 1 tablespoon lemon juice
- ½ cup cilantro, chopped

Directions:

In a pan that fits your air fryer, mix the fish with the other ingredients, toss, introduce in the fryer and cook at 380 degrees F for 15 minutes. Divide everything between plates and serve right away.

Nutrition: calories 220, fat 12, fiber 4, carbs 6, protein 9

Ketogenic Air Fryer Poultry Recipes

Chicken and Cauliflower Rice Casserole
Prep time: 5 minutes | Cooking time: 35 minutes | Servings: 4

Ingredients:

- 2 cups cauliflower florets, chopped
- A pinch of salt and black pepper
- A drizzle of olive oil
- 6 ounces coconut cream
- 2 tablespoons butter, melted
- 2 teaspoons thyme, chopped
- 1 garlic clove, minced
- 1 tablespoon parsley, chopped
- 4 chicken thighs, boneless and skinless

Directions:

Heat up a pan with the butter over medium heat, add the cream and the other ingredients except the cauliflower, oil and the chicken, whisk, bring to a simmer and cook for 5 minutes. Heat up a pan with the oil over medium-high heat, add the chicken and brown for 2 minutes on each side. In a baking dish that fits the air fryer, mix the chicken with the cauliflower, spread the coconut cream mix all over, put the pan in the machine and cook at 380 degrees F for 20 minutes. Divide between plates and serve hot.

Nutrition: calories 280, fat 14, fiber 4, carbs 6, protein 20

Chicken Breasts and Green Beans
Prep time: 5 minutes | Cooking time: 35 minutes | Servings: 4

Ingredients:

- 4 chicken breasts, skinless, boneless and halved
- 10 ounces chicken stock
- 1 teaspoon oregano, dried
- 10 ounces green beans, trimmed and halved
- 2 tablespoons olive oil
- A pinch of salt and black pepper
- 1 tablespoon parsley, chopped

Directions:

Heat up a pan that fits the air fryer with the oil over medium-high heat, add the chicken and brown for 2 minutes on each side. Add the remaining ingredients, toss a bit, put the pan in the machine and cook at 380 degrees F for 30 minutes. Divide everything between plates and serve.

Nutrition: calories 241, fat 11, fiber 5, carbs 6, protein 14

Spring Chicken Mix
Prep time: 5 minutes | Cooking time: 25 minutes | Servings: 4

Ingredients:

- 4 chicken breasts, skinless, boneless and halved
- 2 zucchinis, sliced
- 4 tomatoes, cut into wedges
- 2 yellow bell peppers, cut into wedges
- 2 tablespoons olive oil
- 1 teaspoon Italian seasoning

Directions:

In a baking dish that fits your air fryer, mix all the ingredients, toss, introduce in the fryer and cook at 380 degrees F for 25 minutes. Divide everything between plates and serve.

Nutrition: calories 280, fat 12, fiber 4, carbs 6, protein 14

Spiced Chicken Breasts
Prep time: 5 minutes | Cooking time: 20 minutes | Servings: 4

Ingredients:

- 4 chicken breasts, skinless and boneless
- 1 teaspoon chili powder
- A pinch of salt and black pepper
- A drizzle of olive oil
- 1 teaspoon smoked paprika
- 1 teaspoon garlic powder
- 1 tablespoon parsley, chopped

Directions:

Season chicken with salt and pepper, and rub it with the oil and all the other ingredients except the parsley Put the chicken breasts in your air fryer's basket and cook at 350 degrees F for 10 minutes on each side. Divide between plates, sprinkle the parsley on top and serve.

Nutrition: calories 222, fat 11, fiber 4, carbs 6, protein 12

Roasted Chicken Thighs
Prep time: 5 minutes | Cooking time: 30 minutes | Servings: 4

Ingredients:

- 4 chicken thighs, bone-in and skinless
- A pinch of salt and black pepper
- 1 cup okra
- ½ cup butter, melted
- Zest of 1 lemon, grated
- 4 garlic cloves, minced
- 1 tablespoon thyme, chopped
- 1 tablespoon parsley, chopped

Directions:

Heat up a pan that fits your air fryer with half of the butter over medium heat, add the chicken thighs and brown them for 2-3 minutes on each side. Add the rest of the butter, the okra and all the remaining ingredients, toss, put the pan in the air fryer and cook at 370 degrees F for 20 minutes. Divide between plates and serve.

Nutrition: calories 270, fat 12, fiber 4, carbs 6, protein 14

Crispy Chicken Wings
Prep time: 5 minutes | Cooking time: 30 minutes | Servings: 4

Ingredients:

- 2 pounds chicken wings
- ¼ cup olive oil
- Juice of 2 lemons
- Zest of 1 lemon, grated
- A pinch of salt and black pepper
- 2 garlic cloves, minced

Directions:

In a bowl, mix the chicken wings with the rest of the ingredients and toss well. Put the chicken wings in your air fryer's basket and cook at 400 degrees F for 30 minutes, shaking halfway. Divide between plates and serve with a side salad.

Nutrition: calories 263, fat 14, fiber 4, carbs 6, protein 15

Creamy Chicken Wings
Prep time: 5 minutes | Cooking time: 30 minutes | Servings: 4

Ingredients:
- 2 pounds chicken wings
- Salt and black pepper to the taste
- 3 garlic cloves, minced
- 3 tablespoons butter, melted
- ½ cup heavy cream
- ½ teaspoon basil, dried
- ½ teaspoon oregano, dried
- ¼ cup parmesan, grated

Directions:

In a baking dish that fits your air fryer, mix the chicken wings with all the ingredients except the parmesan and toss. Put the dish to your air fryer and cook at 380 degrees F for 30 minutes. Sprinkle the cheese on top, leave the mix aside for 10 minutes, divide between plates and serve.

Nutrition: calories 270, fat 12, fiber 3, carbs 6, protein 17

Ginger Chicken Breasts
Prep time: 5 minutes | Cooking time: 20 minutes | Servings: 4

Ingredients:
- 4 chicken breasts, skinless, boneless and halved
- 4 tablespoons coconut aminos
- 1 teaspoon olive oil
- 2 tablespoons stevia
- Salt and black pepper to the taste
- ¼ cup chicken stock
- 1 tablespoon ginger, grated

Directions:

In a pan that fits the air fryer, combine the chicken with the ginger and all the ingredients and toss.. Put the pan in your air fryer and cook at 4380 degrees F for 20, shaking the fryer halfway. Divide between plates and serve with a side salad.

Nutrition: calories 256, fat 12, fiber 4, carbs 6, protein 14

Mediterranean Chicken

Prep time: 15 minutes | *Cooking time:* 25 minutes | *Servings:* 4

Ingredients:

- 1 pound chicken thighs, boneless and skinless
- Juice of 1 lemon
- 2 tablespoons olive oil
- 3 garlic cloves, minced
- 1 teaspoon oregano, dried
- ½ pound asparagus, trimmed and halved
- A pinch of salt and black pepper
- 1 zucchinis, halved lengthwise and sliced into half-moons

Directions:

In a bowl, mix the chicken with all the ingredients except the asparagus and the zucchinis, toss and leave aside for 15 minutes. Add the zucchinis and the asparagus, toss, put everything into a pan that fits the air fryer, and cook at 380 degrees F for 25 minutes. Divide everything between plates and serve.

Nutrition: calories 280, fat 11, fiber 4, carbs 6, protein 17

Chicken Thighs and Olives Mix

Prep time: 10 minutes | *Cooking time:* 30 minutes | *Servings:* 4

Ingredients:

- 8 chicken thighs, boneless and skinless
- A pinch of salt and black pepper
- 2 tablespoons olive oil
- 1 teaspoon oregano, dried
- ½ teaspoon garlic powder
- 1 cup pepperoncini, drained and sliced
- ½ cup black olives, pitted and sliced
- ½ cup kalamata olives, pitted and sliced
- ¼ cup parmesan, grated

Directions:

Heat up a pan that fits the air fryer with the oil over medium-high heat, add the chicken and brown for 2 minutes on each side. Add salt, pepper, and all the other ingredients except the parmesan and toss. Put the pan in the air fryer, sprinkle the parmesan on top and cook at 370 degrees F for 25 minutes. Divide the chicken mix between plates and serve.

Nutrition: calories 270, fat 14, fiber 4, carbs 6, protein 18

Chicken Wings and Pesto

Prep time: 10 minutes | Cooking time: 25 minutes | Servings: 4

Ingredients:

- 1 cup basil pesto
- 2 tablespoons olive oil
- A pinch of salt and black pepper
- 1 and ½ pounds chicken wings

Directions:

In a bowl, mix the chicken wings with all the ingredients and toss well. Put the meat in the air fryer's basket and cook at 380 degrees F for 25 minutes. Divide between plates and serve.

Nutrition: calories 244, fat 11, fiber 4, carbs 6, protein 17

Chicken Thighs and Sun-dried Tomatoes

Prep time: 5 minutes | Cooking time: 25 minutes | Servings: 4

Ingredients:

- 4 chicken thighs, skinless, boneless
- 1 tablespoon olive oil
- A pinch of salt and black pepper
- 1 tablespoon thyme, chopped
- 1 cup chicken stock
- 3 garlic cloves, minced
- ½ cup coconut cream
- 1 cup sun-dried tomatoes, chopped
- 4 tablespoons parmesan, grated

Directions:

Heat up a pan that fits the air fryer with the oil over medium-high heat, add the chicken, salt, pepper and the garlic, and brown for 2-3 minutes on each side. Add the rest of the ingredients except the parmesan, toss, put the pan in the air fryer and cook at 370 degrees F for 20 minutes. Sprinkle the parmesan on top, leave the mix aside for 5 minutes, divide everything between plates and serve.

Nutrition: calories 275, fat 12, fiber 4, carbs 6, protein 17

Chicken Drumsticks and Lemon Sauce
Prep time: 5 minutes | Cooking time: 25 minutes | Servings: 4

Ingredients:

- 2 tablespoons spring onions, minced
- 1 tablespoon ginger, grated
- 4 garlic cloves, minced
- 2 tablespoons coconut aminos
- 8 chicken drumsticks
- ½ cup chicken stock
- Salt and black pepper to the taste
- 1 teaspoon olive oil
- ¼ cup cilantro, chopped
- 1 tablespoon lemon juice

Directions:

Heat up a pan with the oil over medium-high heat, add the chicken drumsticks, brown them for 2 minutes on each side and transfer to a pan that fits the fryer. Add all the other ingredients, toss everything, put the pan in the fryer and cook at 370 degrees F for 20 minutes. Divide the chicken and lemon sauce between plates and serve.

Nutrition: calories 267, fat 11, fiber 4, carbs 6, protein 16

Mozzarella Chicken Breasts
Prep time: 5 minutes | Cooking time: 24 minutes | Servings: 6

Ingredients:

- 6 chicken breasts, skinless, boneless and halved
- A pinch of salt and black pepper
- 2 tablespoons olive oil
- 1 pound mozzarella, sliced
- 2 cups baby spinach
- 1 teaspoon Italian seasoning
- 2 tomatoes, sliced
- 1 tablespoon basil, chopped

Directions:

Make slits in each chicken breast halves, season with salt, pepper and Italian seasoning and stuff with mozzarella, spinach and tomatoes. Drizzle the oil over stuffed chicken, put it in your air fryer's basket and cook at 370 degrees F for 12 minutes on each side. Divide between plates and serve with basil sprinkled on top.

Nutrition: calories 285, fat 12, fiber 4, carbs 7, protein 15

Smoked Chicken Wings
Prep time: 5 *minutes* | *Cooking time:* 30 *minutes* | *Servings:* 4

Ingredients:
- 1 tablespoon olive oil
- 2 pounds chicken wings
- 1 tablespoon lime juice
- 2 teaspoons smoked paprika
- 1 teaspoon red pepper flakes, crushed
- Salt and black pepper to the taste

Directions:
In a bowl, mix the chicken wings with all the other ingredients and toss well. Put the chicken wings in your air fryer's basket and cook at 380 degrees F for 15 minutes on each side. Divide between plates and serve with a side salad.

Nutrition: calories 280, fat 13, fiber 3, carbs 6, protein 14

Crispy Chicken Tenders
Prep time: 5 *minutes* | *Cooking time:* 20 *minutes* | *Servings:* 4

Ingredients:
- 4 chicken breasts, skinless, boneless and cut into tenders
- A pinch of salt and black pepper
- 1/3 cup almond flour
- 2 eggs, whisked
- 9 ounces coconut flakes

Directions:
Season the chicken tenders with salt and pepper, dredge them in almond flour, then dip in eggs and roll in coconut flakes. Put the chicken tenders in your air fryer's basket and cook at 400 degrees F for 10 minutes on each side. Divide between plates and serve with a side salad.

Nutrition: calories 250, fat 12, fiber 4, carbs 6, protein 15

Marinated Drumsticks
Prep time: 10 minutes | *Cooking time: 30 minutes* | *Servings: 4*

Ingredients:
- 1 and ½ cups tomato sauce
- 1 teaspoon onion powder
- A pinch of salt and black pepper
- 1 tablespoon coconut aminos
- ½ teaspoon chili powder
- 2 pounds chicken drumsticks

Directions:
In bowl, mix the chicken drumsticks with all the other ingredients, toss and keep in the fridge for 10 minutes. Drain the drumsticks, put them in your air fryer's basket and cook at 380 degrees F for 15 minutes on each side. Divide everything between plates and serve.

Nutrition: calories 254, fat 14, fiber 4, carbs 6, protein 15

Nutmeg Chicken Thighs
Prep time: 5 minutes | *Cooking time: 30 minutes* | *Servings: 4*

Ingredients:
- 2 pounds chicken thighs
- A pinch of salt and black pepper
- 2 tablespoons olive oil
- ½ teaspoon nutmeg, ground

Directions:
Season the chicken thighs with salt and pepper, and rub with the rest of the ingredients. Put the chicken thighs in air fryer's basket, cook at 360 degrees F for 15 minutes on each side, divide between plates and serve.

Nutrition: calories 271, fat 12, fiber 4, carbs 6, protein 13

Chives Chicken Tenders

Prep time: 5 minutes | *Cooking time:* 20 minutes | *Servings:* 4

Ingredients:

- 1 pound chicken tenders, boneless, skinless
- A pinch of salt and black pepper
- Juice of 1 lemon
- 1 tablespoon chives, chopped
- A drizzle of olive oil

Directions:

In a bowl, mix the chicken tenders with all ingredients except the chives, toss, put the meat in your air fryer's basket and cook at 370 degrees F for 10 minutes on each side. Divide between plates and serve with chives sprinkled on top.

Nutrition: calories 230, fat 13, fiber 4, carbs 6, protein 16

Turmeric Chicken Wings Mix

Prep time: 5 minutes | *Cooking time:* 30 minutes | *Servings:* 4

Ingredients:

- 2 pounds chicken wings, halved
- ¼ cup red vinegar
- 4 garlic cloves, minced
- Salt and black pepper to the taste
- 4 tablespoons olive oil
- 1 tablespoon garlic powder
- 1 teaspoon turmeric powder

Directions:

In a bowl, mix the chicken with all the other ingredients and toss well. Put the chicken wings in your air fryer's basket and cook at 370 degrees F for 30 minutes, flipping the meat halfway. Divide everything between plates and serve with a side salad.

Nutrition: calories 250, fat 12, fiber 4, carbs 6, protein 15

Turkey Breasts and Fresh Herbs Mix
Prep time: 10 minutes | Cooking time: 25 minutes | Servings: 4

Ingredients:
- 2 turkey breasts, skinless, boneless and halved
- 4 tablespoons butter, melted
- 2 tablespoons thyme, chopped
- 2 tablespoons sage, chopped
- 1 tablespoons rosemary, chopped
- 2 tablespoons parsley, chopped
- A pinch of salt and black pepper
- 2 cups chicken stock
- 2 celery stalks, chopped

Directions:
Heat up a pan that fits your air fryer with the butter over medium-high heat, add the turkey and brown for 2-3 minutes on each side. Add the herbs, stock, celery, salt and pepper, toss, put the pan in your air fryer, cook at 390 degrees F for 20 minutes. Divide between plates and serve.

Nutrition: calories 284, fat 14, fiber 2, carbs 6, protein 20

Turkey and Rosemary Butter
Prep time: 5 minutes | Cooking time: 24 minutes | Servings: 4

Ingredients:
- 1 turkey breast, skinless, boneless and cut into 4 pieces
- A pinch of salt and black pepper
- Juice of 1 lemon
- 2 tablespoons rosemary, chopped
- 2 tablespoons butter, melted

Directions:
In a bowl, mix the butter with the rosemary, lemon juice, salt and pepper and whisk really well. Brush the turkey pieces with the rosemary butter, put them your air fryer's basket, cook at 380 degrees F for 12 minutes on each side. Divide between plates and serve with a side salad.

Nutrition: calories 236, fat 12, fiber 4, carbs 6, protein 13

Turkey and Shallot Sauce
Prep time: 5 minutes | *Cooking time: 30 minutes* | *Servings: 4*

Ingredients:

- 1 big turkey breast, skinless, boneless and cubed
- 1 tablespoon olive oil
- ¼ teaspoon sweet paprika
- Salt and black pepper to the taste
- 1 cup chicken stock
- 3 tablespoons butter, melted
- 4 shallots, chopped

Directions:

Heat up a pan that fits the air fryer with the olive oil and the butter over medium high heat, add the turkey cubes, and brown for 3 minutes on each side. Add the shallots, stir and sauté for 5 minutes more. Add the paprika, stock, salt and pepper, toss, put the pan in the air fryer and cook at 370 degrees F for 20 minutes. Divide into bowls and serve.

Nutrition: calories 236, fat 12, fiber 4, carbs 6, protein 15

Mustard Turkey Bites
Prep time: 5 minutes | *Cooking time: 20 minutes* | *Servings: 4*

Ingredients:

- 1 big turkey breast, skinless, boneless and cubed
- 4 garlic cloves, minced
- Salt and black pepper to the taste
- 1 and ½ tablespoon olive oil
- 1 tablespoon mustard

Directions:

In a bowl, mix the chicken with the garlic and the other ingredients and toss. Put the turkey in your air fryer's basket, cook at 360 degrees F for 20 minutes, divide between plates and serve with a side salad.

Nutrition: calories 240, fat 12, fiber 4, carbs 6, protein 15

Balsamic Glazed Turkey
Prep time: 5 minutes | Cooking time: 30 minutes | Servings: 4

Ingredients:

- 1 big turkey breast, skinless, boneless and cut into 4 slices
- 3 tablespoons balsamic vinegar
- 2 garlic cloves, minced
- 3 tablespoons butter, melted
- A pinch of salt and black pepper
- 1 tablespoon chives, chopped

Directions:

Heat up a pan that fits the air fryer with the butter over medium-high heat, add the garlic and sauté for 2 minutes. Add the turkey, brown for 2 minutes on each side and take off the heat. Add the rest of the ingredients, toss, put the pan in your air fryer and cook at 380 degrees F for 20 minutes. Divide everything between plates and serve.

Nutrition: calories 283, fat 12, fiber 3, carbs 5, protein 15

Turkey and Gravy
Prep time: 5 minutes | Cooking time: 25 minutes | Servings: 4

Ingredients:

- 1 big turkey breast, skinless, boneless, cubed and browned
- Juice of 1 lime
- Zest of 1 lime, grated
- 1 cup chicken stock
- 3 tablespoons parsley, chopped
- 4 tablespoons butter, melted
- 2 tablespoons thyme, chopped
- A pinch of salt and black pepper

Directions:

Heat up a pan that fits the air fryer with the butter over medium heat, add all the ingredients except the turkey, whisk, bring to a simmer and cook for 5 minutes. Add the turkey cubes, put the pan in the air fryer and cook at 380 degrees F for 20 minutes. Divide the meat between plates, drizzle the gravy all over and serve.

Nutrition: calories 284, fat 13, fiber 3, carbs 5, protein 15

Turkey and Almonds
Prep time: 5 minutes | Cooking time: 25 minutes | Servings: 2

Ingredients:
- 1 big turkey breast, skinless, boneless and halved
- 1/3 cup almonds, chopped
- Salt and black pepper to the taste
- 2 tablespoons olive oil
- 1 tablespoon sweet paprika
- 2 shallots, chopped

Directions:
In a pan that fits the air fryer, combine the turkey with all the other ingredients, toss, put the pan in the machine and cook at 370 degrees F for 25 minutes. Divide everything between plates and serve.

Nutrition: calories 274, fat 12, fiber 3, carbs 5, protein 14

Turkey Strips and Leeks
Prep time: 5 minutes | Cooking time: 30 minutes | Servings: 4

Ingredients:
- 1 turkey breast, skinless, boneless and cut into strips
- A pinch of salt and black pepper
- 1 tablespoon olive oil
- 1 cup veggie stock
- 4 leeks, sliced
- 2 tablespoon chives, chopped

Directions:
Heat up a pan that fits your air fryer with the oil over medium heat, add the meat and brown for 2 minutes on each side. Add the remaining ingredients, toss, put the pan in the machine and cook at 380 degrees F for 25 minutes. Divide everything between plates and serve with a side salad.

Nutrition: calories 257, fat 12, fiber 4, carbs 5, protein 14

Turkey and Cherry Tomatoes Pan
Prep time: 5 minutes | Cooking time: 25 minutes | Servings: 4

Ingredients:
- 1 pound turkey breast, skinless, boneless and cubed
- 1 cup heavy cream
- A pinch of salt and black pepper
- 4 ounces cherry tomatoes, halved
- 1 tablespoon ginger, grated
- 2 tablespoons red chili powder
- 2 teaspoons olive oil

Directions:
Heat up a pan that fits the air fryer with the oil over medium heat, add the turkey and brown for 2 minutes on each side. Add the rest of the ingredients, toss, put the pan in the machine and cook at 380 degrees F for 20 minutes. Divide everything between plates and serve.

Nutrition: calories 267, fat 13, fiber 4, carbs 6, protein 16

Turkey Breasts and Celery
Prep time: 5 minutes | Cooking time: 30 minutes | Servings: 4

Ingredients:
- 1 big turkey breast, skinless, boneless and sliced
- 4 garlic cloves, minced
- 3 tablespoons olive oil
- 4 celery stalks, roughly chopped
- 1 teaspoon turmeric powder
- 1 teaspoon cumin, ground
- 1 tablespoon smoked paprika
- 1 tablespoon garlic powder

Directions:
In a pan that fits the air fryer, combine the turkey and the other ingredients, toss, put the pan in the machine and cook at 380 degrees F for 30 minutes. Divide everything between plates and serve.

Nutrition: calories 285, fat 12, fiber 3, carbs 6, protein 16

Turkey and Mushroom Sauce

Preparation time: 5 minutes
Cooking time: 25 minutes
Servings: 4

Ingredients:

- 6 cups leftover turkey meat, skinless, boneless and shredded
- A pinch of salt and black pepper
- 1 tablespoon parsley, chopped
- 1 cup chicken stock
- 3 tablespoons butter, melted
- 1 pound mushrooms, sliced
- 2 spring onions, chopped

Directions:

Heat up a pan that fits the air fryer with the butter over medium-high heat, add the mushrooms and sauté for 5 minutes. Add the rest of the ingredients, toss, put the pan in the machine and cook at 370 degrees F for 20 minutes. Divide everything between plates and serve.

Nutrition: calories 285, fat 11, fiber 3, carbs 5, protein 14

Turkey and Spinach Mix
Prep time: 5 minutes | Cooking time: 15 minutes | Servings: 4

Ingredients:

- 1 pound turkey meat, ground and browned
- 1 tablespoon garlic, minced
- 1 tablespoon ginger, grated
- 2 tablespoons coconut aminos
- 4 cups spinach leaves
- A pinch of salt and black pepper

Directions:

In a pan that fits your air fryer, combine all the ingredients and toss. Put the pan in the air fryer and cook at 380 degrees F for 15 minutes Divide everything into bowls and serve.

Nutrition: calories 240, fat 12, fiber 3, carbs 5, protein 13

Turkey and Asparagus
Prep time: 5 minutes | Cooking time: 25 minutes | Servings: 4

Ingredients:
- 1 pound turkey breast tenderloins, cut into strips
- 1 pound asparagus, trimmed and cut into medium pieces
- A pinch of salt and black pepper
- 1 tablespoon lemon juice
- 1 teaspoon coconut aminos
- 2 tablespoons olive oil
- 2 garlic cloves, minced
- ¼ cup chicken stock

Directions:
Heat up a pan that fits the air fryer with the oil over medium-high heat, add the meat and brown for 2 minutes on each side. Add the rest of the ingredients, toss, put the pan in the machine and cook at 380 degrees F for 20 minutes. Divide everything between plates and serve

Nutrition: calories 264, fat 14, fiber 4, carbs 6, protein 16

Ground Turkey and Green Beans
Prep time: 5 minutes | Cooking time: 25 minutes | Servings: 4

Ingredients:
- 1 pound turkey meat, ground
- A pinch of salt and black pepper
- 2 tablespoons olive oil
- 2 teaspoons parsley flakes
- 1 pound green beans, trimmed and halved
- 2 teaspoons garlic powder

Directions:
Heat up a pan that fits the air fryer with the oil over medium-high heat, add the meat and brown it for 5 minutes. Add the remaining ingredients, toss, put the pan in the machine and cook at 370 degrees F for 20 minutes. Divide between plates and serve.

Nutrition: calories 274, fat 12, fiber 3, carbs 6, protein 15

Turkey and Red Cabbage Pan
Prep time: 5 minutes | *Cooking time:* 25 minutes | *Servings:* 4

Ingredients:

- 1 pound turkey meat, ground
- A pinch of salt and black pepper
- 2 tablespoons butter, melted
- 1 ounce chicken stock
- 1 small red cabbage head, shredded
- 1 tablespoon sweet paprika, chopped
- 1 tablespoon parsley, chopped

Directions:

Heat up a pan that fits the air fryer with the butter, add the meat and brown for 5 minutes. Add all the other ingredients, toss, put the pan in the air fryer and cook at 380 degrees F for 20 minutes. Divide everything between plates and serve.

Nutrition: calories 284, fat 13, fiber 4, carbs 5, protein 14

Cheddar Turkey Bites
Prep time: 5 minutes | *Cooking time:* 20 minutes | *Servings:* 4

Ingredients:

- 1 big turkey breast, skinless, boneless and cubed
- Salt and black pepper to the taste
- ¼ cup cheddar cheese, grated
- ¼ teaspoon garlic powder
- 1 tablespoon olive oil

Directions:

Rub the turkey cubes with the oil, season with salt, pepper and garlic powder and dredge in cheddar cheese. Put the turkey bits in your air fryer's basket and cook at 380 degrees F for 20 minutes. Divide between plates and serve with a side salad.

Nutrition: calories 240, fat 11, fiber 2, carbs 5, protein 12

Ground Turkey and Broccoli
Prep time: *5 minutes* | ***Cooking time:*** *25 minutes* | ***Servings:*** *4*

Ingredients:
- 1 pound turkey meat, ground
- 2 garlic cloves, minced
- 1 teaspoon ginger, grated
- 2 teaspoons coconut aminos
- 3 tablespoons olive oil
- 2 broccoli heads, florets separated and then halved
- A pinch of salt and black pepper
- 1 teaspoon chili paste

Directions:
Heat up a pan that fits the air fryer with the oil over medium heat, add the meat and brown for 5 minutes. Add the rest of the ingredients, toss, put the pan in the fryer and cook at 380 degrees F for 20 minutes. Divide everything between plates and serve.

Nutrition: calories 274, fat 11, fiber 3, carbs 6, protein 12

Turkey and Kale
Prep time: *5 minutes* | ***Cooking time:*** *25 minutes* | ***Servings:*** *4*

Ingredients:
- 1 pound turkey meat, ground
- A pinch of salt and black pepper
- 2 tablespoons olive oil
- 1 teaspoon coconut aminos
- 2 spring onions, minced
- 4 cups kale, chopped
- 1 tablespoon garlic, chopped
- 1 red chili pepper, chopped
- ½ cup chicken stock

Directions:
Heat up a pan that fits your air fryer with the oil over medium heat, add the meat, salt, pepper, spring onions and the garlic, stir and sauté for 5 minutes. Add the rest of the ingredients, toss, put the pan in the fryer and cook at 380 degrees F for 20 minutes. Divide between plates and serve

Nutrition: calories 261, fat 12, fiber 2, carbs 5, protein 13

Cumin Turkey Mix
Prep time: 5 minutes | *Cooking time: 25 minutes* | *Servings: 4*

Ingredients:

- 1 pound turkey meat, cubed and browned
- A pinch of salt and black pepper
- 1 green bell pepper, chopped
- 3 garlic cloves, chopped
- 1 and ½ teaspoons cumin, ground
- 12 ounces veggies stock
- 1 cup tomatoes, chopped

Directions:

In a pan that fits your air fryer, mix the turkey with the rest of the ingredients, toss, put the pan in the machine and cook at 380 degrees F for 25 minutes. Divide into bowls and serve.

Nutrition: calories 274, fat 12, fiber 4, carbs 6, protein 15

Oregano Turkey Bowls
Prep time: 5 minutes | *Cooking time: 25 minutes* | *Servings: 4*

Ingredients:

- 1 pound turkey meat, ground
- Salt and black pepper to the taste
- 2 tablespoons olive oil
- 10 ounces tomato sauce
- 1 tablespoon oregano, chopped
- 2 cups spinach

Directions:

Heat up a pan that fits your air fryer with the oil over medium heat, add the turkey, oregano, salt and pepper, stir and brown for 5 minutes. Add the tomato sauce, toss, put the pan in the machine and cook at 370 degrees F for 15 minutes. Add spinach, toss, cook for 5 minutes more, divide everything into bowls and serve.

Nutrition: calories 263, fat 12, fiber 3, carbs 6, protein 16

Duck and Mushroom Rice
Prep time: *5 minutes* | ***Cooking time:*** *20 minutes* | ***Servings:*** *4*

Ingredients:
- 2 ounces mushrooms, sliced
- 2 tablespoons olive oil
- 2 cups cauliflower florets, riced
- ½ cup walnuts, toasted and chopped
- 2 cups chicken stock
- A pinch of salt and black pepper
- ½ cup parsley, chopped
- 2 pounds duck breasts, boneless and skin scored

Directions:
Heat up a pan that fits the air fryer with the oil over medium-high heat, add the duck breasts skin side down and brown for 4 minutes. Add the mushrooms, cauliflower, salt and pepper, and cook for 1 minute more. Add the stock, introduce the pan in the air fryer and cook at 380 degrees F for 15 minutes. Divide the mix between plates, sprinkle the parsley and walnuts on top and serve.

Nutrition: calories 268, fat 12, fiber 4, carbs 6, protein 17

Duck Breast and Blackberry Sauce
Prep time: *5 minutes* | ***Cooking time:*** *25 minutes* | ***Servings:*** *4*

Ingredients:
- 4 duck breasts, boneless and skin scored
- A pinch of salt and black pepper
- 2 tablespoons olive oil
- 1 and ½ cups chicken stock
- 2 spring onions, chopped
- 4 garlic cloves, minced
- 1 and ½ cups blackberries, pureed
- 2 tablespoons butter, melted

Directions:
Heat up a pan that fits the air fryer with the oil and the butter over medium-high heat, add the duck breasts skin side down and sear for 5 minutes. Add the remaining ingredients, toss, put the pan in the air fryer and cook at 370 degrees F for 20 minutes. Divide the duck and sauce between plates and serve.

Nutrition: calories 265, fat 14, fiber 3, carbs 5, protein 14

Spiced Duck Legs
Prep time: 5 minutes | *Cooking time:* 25 minutes | *Servings:* 4

Ingredients:
- 4 duck legs
- 2 garlic cloves, minced
- 1 teaspoon five spice
- A pinch of salt and black pepper
- 2 tablespoons olive oil
- 1 teaspoon hot chili powder

Directions:
In a bowl, mix the duck legs with all the other ingredients and rub them well. Put the duck legs in your air fryer's basket and cook at 380 degrees F for 25 minutes, flipping them halfway. Divide between plates and serve.

Nutrition: calories 287, fat 12, fiber 4, carbs 6, protein 17

Thyme Duck Legs
Prep time: 5 minutes | *Cooking time:* 30 minutes | *Servings:* 4

Ingredients:
- 4 duck legs
- A pinch of salt and black pepper
- 3 teaspoons fennel seeds, crushed
- 4 teaspoons thyme, dried
- 2 tablespoons olive oil

Directions:
In a bowl, mix the duck legs with all the other ingredients and toss well. Put the duck legs in your air fryer's basket and cook at 380 degrees F for 15 minutes on each side. Divide between plates and serve

Nutrition: calories 274, fat 11, fiber 4, carbs 6, protein 14

Cinnamon Duck Breasts

Prep time: 5 minutes | Cooking time: 20 minutes | Servings: 2

Ingredients:

- 2 duck breasts, boneless and skin scored
- A pinch of salt and black pepper
- ¼ teaspoon cinnamon powder
- 4 tablespoons stevia
- 3 tablespoons balsamic vinegar

Directions:

In a bowl, mix the duck breasts with the rest of the ingredients and rub well. Put the duck breasts in your air fryer's basket and cook at 380 degrees F for 10 minutes on each side. Divide everything between plates and serve.

Nutrition: calories 294, fat 12, fiber 4, carbs 6, protein 15

Cardamom Duck Legs

Prep time: 5 minutes | Cooking time: 30 minutes | Servings: 4

Ingredients:

- 4 duck legs
- Juice of ½ lemon
- Zest of ½ lemon, grated
- 1 tablespoon cardamom, crushed
- ¼ teaspoon allspice
- 2 tablespoons almonds, toasted and chopped
- 2 tablespoons olive oil

Directions:

In a bowl, mix the duck legs with the remaining ingredients except the almonds and toss. Put the duck legs in your air fryer's basket and cook at 380 degrees F for 15 minutes on each side. Divide the duck legs between plates, sprinkle the almonds on top and serve with a side salad.

Nutrition: calories 284, fat 12, fiber 4, carbs 6, protein 18

Duck with Cinnamon and Olives
Prep time: 5 minutes | Cooking time: 25 minutes | Servings: 2

Ingredients:
- 2 duck legs
- 1 teaspoon cinnamon powder
- 1 tablespoon olive oil
- 1 garlic clove, minced
- A pinch of salt and black pepper
- 2 ounces black olives, pitted and sliced
- Juice of ½ lime
- 1 tablespoon parsley, chopped

Directions:
In a bowl, mix the duck legs with cinnamon, oil, garlic, salt and pepper, and rub well. Heat up a pan that fits the air fryer over medium-high heat, add duck legs and brown for 2-3 minutes on each side. Add the remaining ingredients to the pan, put the pan in the air fryer and cook at 400 degrees F for 10 minutes on each side. Divide between plates and serve.

Nutrition: calories 276, fat 12, fiber 4, carbs 6, protein 14

Vanilla Duck Legs
Prep time: 5 minutes | Cooking time: 30 minutes | Servings: 4

Ingredients:
- 4 duck legs, skin on
- Juice of ½ lemon
- 1 teaspoon cinnamon powder
- 1 teaspoon vanilla extract
- 10 peppercorns, crushed
- 1 tablespoon balsamic vinegar
- 1 tablespoon olive oil
- A pinch of salt and black pepper

Directions:
Heat up a pan with the oil over medium-high heat, add the duck legs and sear them for 3 minutes on each side. Transfer to a pan that fits the air fryer, add the remaining ingredients, toss, put the pan in the air fryer and cook at 380 degrees F for 22 minutes. Divide duck legs and cooking juices between plates and serve.

Nutrition: calories 271, fat 13, fiber 4, carbs 6, protein 15

Duck Breast and Veggies
Prep time: 5 minutes | Cooking time: 25 minutes | Servings: 6

Ingredients:

- 6 duck breasts, boneless, skin on and scored
- 1 tablespoon balsamic vinegar
- 1 tablespoon coconut aminos
- A pinch of salt and black pepper
- 2 courgettes, sliced
- ¼ pound oyster mushrooms, sliced
- ½ bunch coriander, chopped
- 2 tablespoons olive oil
- 3 garlic cloves, minced

Directions:

Heat up a pan that fits your air fryer with the oil over medium heat, add the duck breasts skin side down and sear for 5 minutes. Add the rest of the ingredients, cook for 2 minutes more, transfer the pan to the air fryer and cook at 380 degrees F for 20 minutes. Divide everything between plates and serve.

Nutrition: calories 2764, fat 12, fiber 4, carbs 6, protein 14

Duck Breast and Peppers Sauce
Prep time: 5 minutes | Cooking time: 25 minutes | Servings: 4

Ingredients:

- 4 duck breast fillets, skin-on
- 1 tablespoon balsamic vinegar
- 4 tablespoons olive oil
- 1 red bell pepper, roasted, peeled and chopped
- 1/3 cup basil, chopped
- 1 tablespoon pine nuts
- 1 teaspoon tarragon
- 1 garlic clove, minced
- 1 tablespoon lemon juice

Directions:

Heat up a pan that fist your air fryer with half of the oil over medium heat, add the duck fillets skin side up and cook for 2-3 minutes. Add the vinegar, toss and cook for 2 minutes more. In a blender, combine the rest of the oil with the remaining ingredients and pulse well. Pour this over the duck, put the pan in the fryer and cook at 370 degrees F for 16 minutes. Divide everything between plates and serve.

Nutrition: calories 270, fat 14, fiber 3, carbs 6, protein 16

Duck and Eggplant Mix
Prep time: 5 minutes | Cooking time: 25 minutes | Servings: 4

Ingredients:
- 1 pound duck breasts, skinless, boneless and cubed
- 2 eggplants, cubed
- A pinch of salt and black pepper
- 2 tablespoons olive oil
- 1 tablespoon sweet paprika
- ½ cup tomato sauce

Directions:
Heat up a pan that fits your air fryer with the oil over medium heat, add the duck pieces and brown for 5 minutes. Add the rest of the ingredients, toss, introduce the pan in the fryer and cook at 370 degrees F for 20 minutes. Divide between plates and serve.

Nutrition: calories 285, fat 14, fiber 4, carbs 6, protein 16

Creamy Duck Mix
Prep time: 5 minutes | Cooking time: 25 minutes | Servings: 4

Ingredients:
- 15 ounces duck breasts, skinless, boneless and cubed
- 1 tablespoon olive oil
- 2 shallots, chopped
- Salt and black pepper to the taste
- 5 ounces heavy cream
- 1 teaspoon curry powder
- ½ bunch coriander, chopped

Directions:
Heat up a pan that fits your air fryer with the oil over medium heat, add the duck, toss and brown for 5 minutes. Add the rest of the ingredients, toss, introduce the pan in the air fryer and cook at 370 degrees F for 20 minutes. Divide the mix into bowls and serve.

Nutrition: calories 274, fat 14, fiber 4, carbs 7, protein 16

Duck, Peppers and Asparagus Mix
Prep time: 5 minutes | Cooking time: 25 minutes | Servings: 4

Ingredients:
- 2 duck breast fillets, boneless
- ½ cup tomato sauce
- A drizzle of olive oil
- Salt and black pepper to the taste
- 1 cup red bell pepper, chopped
- ½ pound asparagus, trimmed and halved
- ½ cup cheddar cheese, grated

Directions:
Heat up a pan that fits your air fryer with the oil over medium heat, add the duck fillets and brown for 5 minutes. Add the rest of the ingredients except the cheese, toss, put the pan in the air fryer and cook at 370 degrees F for 20 minutes. Sprinkle the cheese on top, divide the mix between plates and serve.

Nutrition: calories 263, fat 12, fiber 4, carbs 6, protein 14

Duck Salad
Prep time: 5 minutes | Cooking time: 20 minutes | Servings: 4

Ingredients:
- 2 duck breasts, boneless and skin on
- 1 teaspoon coconut oil, melted
- A pinch of salt and black pepper
- 2 shallots, sliced
- 12 cherry tomatoes, halved
- 1 tablespoon balsamic vinegar
- 3 cups lettuce leaves, torn
- 12 mint leaves, torn

For the dressing:
- 1 tablespoon lemon juice
- ½ tablespoon balsamic vinegar
- 2 and ½ tablespoons olive oil
- ½ teaspoon mustard

Directions:
Heat up a pan that fits your air fryer with the coconut oil over medium heat, add the duck breasts skin side down and cook for 3 minutes. Add salt, pepper, shallots, tomatoes and 1 tablespoon balsamic vinegar, toss, put the pan in the fryer and cook at 370 degrees F for 17 minutes. Cool this mix down, thinly slice the duck breast and put it along with the tomatoes and shallots in a bowl. Add mint and salad leaves and toss. In a separate bowl, mix ½ tablespoon vinegar with lemon juice, oil and mustard and whisk well. Pour this over the duck salad, toss and serve.

Nutrition: calories 241, fat 10, fiber 2, carbs 5, protein 15

Duck Breast and Cranberry Sauce
Prep time: 5 minutes | Cooking time: 25 minutes | Servings: 4

Ingredients:
- 4 duck breasts, boneless, skin-on and scored
- A pinch of salt and black pepper
- 1 tablespoon olive oil
- ¼ cup balsamic vinegar
- ½ cup dried cranberries

Directions:
Heat up a pan that fits your air fryer with the oil over medium-high heat, add the duck breasts skin side down and cook for 5 minutes. Add the rest of the ingredients, toss, put the pan in the fryer and cook at 380 degrees F for 20 minutes. Divide between plates and serve.

Nutrition: calories 287, fat 12, fiber 4, carbs 6, protein 16

Parsley Duck Breast Mix
Prep time: 10 minutes | Cooking time: 25 minutes | Servings: 4

Ingredients:
- 4 duck breast fillets, boneless, skin-on and scored
- 2 tablespoons olive oil
- 2 tablespoons parsley, chopped
- Salt and black pepper to the taste
- 1 cup chicken stock
- 1 teaspoon balsamic vinegar

Directions:
Heat up a pan that fits your air fryer with the oil over medium heat, add the duck breasts skin side down and sear for 5 minutes. Add the rest of the ingredients, toss, put the pan in the fryer and cook at 380 degrees F for 20 minutes. Divide everything between plates and serve

Nutrition: calories 274, fat 14, fiber 4, carbs 6, protein 16

Basil Duck
Prep time: 5 minutes | Cooking time: 25 minutes | Servings: 4

Ingredients:
- 3 garlic cloves, minced
- 4 duck breasts, boneless, skin-on and scored
- 2 tablespoons olive oil
- ¼ teaspoon coriander, ground
- 14 ounces coconut milk
- Salt and black pepper to the taste
- 1 cup basil, chopped

Directions:
Heat up a pan that fits your air fryer with the oil over medium heat, add the duck breasts, skin side down and sear for 5 minutes. Add the rest of the ingredients, toss, put the pan in the fryer and cook at 380 degrees F for 20 minutes. Divide between plates and serve.

Nutrition: calories 274, fat 13, fiber 3, carbs 5, protein 16

Creamy Duck and Tomatoes Mix
Prep time: 5 minutes | Cooking time: 25 minutes | Servings: 4

Ingredients:
- 1 yellow onion, chopped
- 2 tablespoons butter, melted
- 4 garlic cloves, minced
- 1 and ½ teaspoons coriander, ground
- Salt and black pepper to the taste
- 15 ounces canned tomatoes, crushed
- ¼ cup lemon juice
- 1 and ½ pounds duck breast, skinless, boneless and cubed
- ½ cup cilantro, chopped
- ½ cup chicken stock
- ½ cup heavy cream

Directions:
Heat up a pan that fits your air fryer with the butter over medium heat, add the duck pieces and cook for 5 minutes. Add the rest of the ingredients except the cilantro, toss, introduce the pan in the fryer and cook at 370 degrees F for 20 minutes. Divide between plates and serve.

Nutrition: calorie 284, fat 12, fiber 4, carbs 6, protein 17

Sesame Chicken Mix
Prep time: 10 minutes | Cooking time: 20 minutes | Servings: 4

Ingredients:

- 2 pounds duck breast, skinless, boneless and cubed
- ½ cup spring onions, chopped
- Salt and black pepper to the taste
- 1 tablespoon olive oil
- 2 garlic cloves, minced
- ¼ teaspoon red pepper flakes, crushed
- 1 tablespoons sesame seeds, toasted

Directions:

Heat up a pan that fits your air fryer with the oil over medium heat, add the meat, toss and brown for 5 minutes. Add the rest of the ingredients except the sesame seeds, toss, introduce in the fryer and cook at 380 degrees F for 15 minutes. Add sesame seeds, toss, divide between plates and serve.

Nutrition: calories 264, fat 12, fiber 4, carbs 6, protein 17

Thyme and Paprika Duck
Prep time: 5 minutes | Cooking time: 25 minutes | Servings: 4

Ingredients:

- 1 pound duck breasts, skinless, boneless and cubed
- Salt and black pepper to the taste
- 1 tablespoon olive oil
- ½ teaspoon sweet paprika
- ¼ cup chicken stock
- 1 teaspoon thyme, chopped

Directions:

Heat up a pan that fits your air fryer with the oil over medium heat, add the duck pieces, and brown them for 5 minutes. Add the rest of the ingredients, toss, put the pan in the machine and cook at 380 degrees F for 20 minutes. Divide between plates and serve.

Nutrition: calories 264, fat 14, fiber 4, carbs 6, protein 18

Ketogenic Air Fryer Meat Recipes

Pork Tenderloin and Veggies
Prep time: 5 minutes | Cooking time: 25 minutes | Servings: 4

Ingredients:

- 1 pound pork tenderloin, sliced
- ¼ cup cilantro, chopped
- ½ teaspoon garlic powder
- 1 tablespoon olive oil
- 1 green bell pepper, julienned
- ½ teaspoon chili powder
- ½ teaspoon cumin, ground

Directions:

Heat up a pan that fits the air fryer with the oil over medium heat, add the pork and brown for 5 minutes. Add the rest of the ingredients, toss, put the pan in the air fryer and cook at 400 degrees F for 20 minutes. Divide between plates and serve.

Nutrition: calories 284, fat 13, fiber 4, carbs 6, protein 17

Paprika Pork Mix
Prep time: 5 minutes | Cooking time: 25 minutes | Servings: 4

Ingredients:

- 1 pound pork stew meat, cubed
- 4 teaspoons sweet paprika
- A pinch of salt and black pepper
- 1 cup coconut cream
- 1 tablespoon butter, melted
- 1 tablespoon parsley, chopped

Directions:

Heat up a pan that fits the air fryer with the butter over medium heat, add the meat and brown for 5 minutes. Add the remaining ingredients, toss, put the pan in the air fryer, cook at 390 degrees F for 20 minutes more, divide into bowls and serve.

Nutrition: calories 273, fat 12, fiber 4, carbs 6, protein 20

Smoked Pork Chops
Prep time: *5 minutes* | ***Cooking time:*** *25 minutes* | ***Servings:*** *4*

Ingredients:
- 4 pork chops
- 1 tablespoon smoked paprika
- 1 tablespoon olive oil
- 2 tablespoons balsamic vinegar
- ½ cup chicken stock
- A pinch of salt and black pepper

Directions:
In a bowl, mix the pork chops with the rest of the ingredients and toss. Put the pork chops in your air fryer's basket and cook at 390 degrees F for 25 minutes. Divide between plates and serve.

Nutrition: calories 276, fat 12, fiber 4, carbs 6, protein 22

Mustard Pork Chops
Prep time: *5 minutes* | ***Cooking time:*** *25 minutes* | ***Servings:*** *4*

Ingredients:
- 4 pork chops
- A pinch of salt and black pepper
- 2/3 cup cream cheese, soft
- ¼ teaspoon garlic powder
- 10 ounces beef stock
- ¼ teaspoon oregano, dried
- 1 tablespoon mustard
- ¼ teaspoon thyme, dried
- 1 tablespoon olive oil
- 1 tablespoon parsley, chopped

Directions:
In a baking dish that fits your air fryer, mix all the ingredients, introduce the pan in the fryer and cook at 400 degrees F for 25 minutes. Divide everything between plates and serve.

Nutrition: calories 284, fat 14, fiber 4, carbs 6, protein 22

Vinegar Pork Chops
Prep time: 5 minutes | Cooking time: 25 minutes | Servings: 4

Ingredients:
- 2 tablespoons olive oil
- 4 pork chops
- A pinch of salt and black pepper
- 4 garlic cloves, minced
- 3 tablespoons cider vinegar

Directions:
Heat up a pan that fits the air fryer with the oil over medium-high heat, add the pork chops and brown for 5 minutes. Add the rest of the ingredients, toss, put the pan in your air fryer and cook at 400 degrees F for 20 minutes. Divide between plates and serve.

Nutrition: calories 273, fat 13, fiber 4, carbs 6, protein 22

Pork Medallions and Garlic Sauce
Prep time: 5 minutes | Cooking time: 25 minutes | Servings: 4

Ingredients:
- 1 pound pork tenderloin, sliced
- A pinch of salt and black pepper
- 4 tablespoons butter, melted
- 2 teaspoons garlic, minced
- 1 teaspoon sweet paprika

Directions:
Heat up a pan that fits the air fryer with the butter over medium heat, add all the ingredients except the pork medallions, whisk well and simmer for 4-5 minutes. Add the pork, toss, put the pan in your air fryer and cook at 380 degrees F for 20 minutes. Divide between plates and serve with a side salad.

Nutrition: calories 284, fat 12, fiber 4, carbs 6, protein 19

Coconut and Chili Pork
Prep time: 5 *minutes* | *Cooking time:* 25 *minutes* | *Servings:* 4

Ingredients:
- 2 teaspoons chili paste
- 2 garlic cloves, minced
- 4 pork chops
- 1 shallot, chopped
- 1 and ½ cups coconut milk
- 2 tablespoons olive oil
- 3 tablespoons coconut aminos
- Salt and black pepper to the taste

Directions:

In a pan that fits your air fryer, mix the pork the rest of the ingredients, toss, introduce the pan in the fryer and cook at 400 degrees F for 25 minutes, shaking the fryer halfway. Divide everything into bowls and serve.

Nutrition: calories 267, fat 12, fiber 4, carbs 6, protein 18

Basil Pork Chops
Prep time: 5 *minutes* | *Cooking time:* 25 *minutes* | *Servings:* 4

Ingredients:
- 4 pork chops
- A pinch of salt and black pepper
- 2 teaspoons basil, dried
- 2 tablespoons olive oil
- ½ teaspoon chili powder

Directions:

In a pan that fits your air fryer, mix all the ingredients, toss, introduce in the fryer and cook at 400 degrees F for 25 minutes. Divide everything between plates and serve.

Nutrition: calories 274, fat 13, fiber 4, carbs 6, protein 18

Pork Chops and Tomato Sauce
Prep time: 5 minutes | Cooking time: 25 minutes | Servings: 4

Ingredients:
- 1 tablespoon mustard
- ¼ cup tomato sauce
- 4 pork chops
- A pinch of salt and black pepper
- 1 teaspoon garlic powder
- 2 teaspoons smoked paprika
- 1 and ½ teaspoons peppercorns, crushed
- A pinch of cayenne pepper
- A drizzle of olive oil

Directions:
Heat up a pan that fits your air fryer with the oil over medium heat, add the pork chops and brown for 5 minutes. Add the rest of the ingredients, toss, put the pan in the fryer and cook at 400 degrees F for 20 minutes. Divide everything between plates and serve.

Nutrition: calories 280, fat 13, fiber 4, carbs 6, protein 18

Pork with Lemon Sauce
Prep time: 15 minutes | Cooking time: 25 minutes | Servings: 4

Ingredients:
- 4 pork chops
- 2 tablespoons olive oil
- A pinch of salt and black pepper
- 2 garlic cloves, minced
- 4 teaspoons mustard
- 2 teaspoons lemon zest, grated
- Juice of 1 lemon

Directions:
In a bowl, mix the pork chops with the other ingredients, toss and keep in the fridge for 15 minutes Put the pork chops in your air fryer's basket and cook at 390 degrees F for 25 minutes. Divide between plates and serve with a side salad.

Nutrition: calories 287, fat 13, fiber 4, carbs 6, protein 20

Pork Roast
Prep time: 5 minutes | Cooking time: 30 minutes | Servings: 4

Ingredients:
- 1 pound pork tenderloin, trimmed
- A pinch of salt and black pepper
- 2 tablespoons olive oil
- 3 tablespoons mustard
- 2 tablespoons balsamic vinegar

Directions:
In a bowl, mix the pork tenderloin with the rest of the ingredients and rub well. Put the roast in your air fryer's basket and cook at 380 degrees F for 30 minutes. Slice the roast, divide between plates and serve.

Nutrition: calories 274, fat 13, fiber 4, carbs 7, protein 22

Pork and Green Beans
Prep time: 5 minutes | Cooking time: 25 minutes | Servings: 4

Ingredients:
- 4 pork chops
- 2 tablespoons coconut oil, melted
- 2 garlic cloves, minced
- A pinch of salt and black pepper
- ½ pound green beans, trimmed and halved
- 2 tablespoons tomato sauce

Directions:
Heat up a pan that fits the air fryer with the oil over medium heat, add the pork chops and brown for 5 minutes. Add the rest of the ingredients, put the pan in the machine and cook at 390 degrees F for 20 minutes. Divide everything between plates and serve

Nutrition: calories 284, fat 13, fiber 4, carbs 6, protein 22

Greek Pork and Cheese
Prep time: 5 minutes | Cooking time: 25 minutes | Servings: 4

Ingredients:

- 2 pounds pork tenderloin, cut into strips
- 2 tablespoons coconut oil, melted
- A pinch of salt and black pepper
- 6 ounces baby spinach
- 1 cup cherry tomatoes, halved
- 1 cup feta cheese, crumbled

Directions:

Heat up a pan that fits your air fryer with the oil over medium high heat, add the pork and brown for 5 minutes. Add the rest of the ingredients except the spinach and the cheese, put the pan to your air fryer, cook at 390 degrees F for 15 minutes. Add the spinach, toss, and cook for 5 minutes more. Divide between plates and serve with feta cheese sprinkled on top.

Nutrition: calories 284, fat 12, fiber 4, carbs 7, protein 22

Oregano Pork and Asparagus
Prep time: 5 minutes | Cooking time: 35 minutes | Servings: 4

Ingredients:

- 2 pounds pork loin, boneless and cubed
- ¾ cup beef stock
- 2 tablespoons olive oil
- 3 tablespoons tomato sauce
- 1 pound asparagus, trimmed and halved
- ½ tablespoon oregano, chopped
- Salt and black pepper to the taste

Directions:

Heat up a pan that fits your air fryer with the oil over medium heat, add the pork, toss and brown for 5 minutes. Add the rest of the ingredients, toss a bit, put the pan in the fryer and cook at 380 degrees F for 30 minutes. Divide everything between plates and serve.

Nutrition: calories 287, fat 13, fiber 4, carbs 6, protein 18

Chipotle Pork Chops
Prep time: 5 minutes | Cooking time: 35 minutes | Servings: 4

Ingredients:
- 4 pork chops, bone-in
- A pinch of salt and black pepper
- 2 and ½ tablespoons ghee, melted
- ½ teaspoon chipotle chili powder
- ½ teaspoon cinnamon powder
- ½ teaspoon garlic powder
- ½ teaspoon allspice
- 1 teaspoon coconut sugar

Directions:

Rub the pork chops with all the other ingredients, put them in your air fryer's basket and cook at 380 degrees F for 35 minutes. Divide the chops between plates and serve with a side salad.

Nutrition: calories 287, fat 14, fiber 4, carbs 7, protein 18

Pork and Bok Choy
Prep time: 5 minutes | Cooking time: 35 minutes | Servings: 4

Ingredients:
- 4 pork chops, boneless
- 1 bok choy head, torn
- 2 cups chicken stock
- 2 tablespoons coconut aminos
- 2 garlic cloves, minced
- A pinch of salt and black pepper
- 2 tablespoons coconut oil, melted

Directions:

Heat up a pan that fits the air fryer with the oil over medium-high heat, add the pork chops and brown for 5 minutes. Add the garlic, salt and pepper and cook for another minute. Add the rest of the ingredients except the bok choy and cook at 380 degrees F for 25 minutes. Add the bok choy, cook for 5 minutes more, divide everything between plates and serve.

Nutrition: calories 284, fat 14, fiber 4, carbs 6, protein 17

Cajun Pork Mix

Prep time: 5 *minutes* | *Cooking time:* 35 *minutes* | *Servings:* 2

Ingredients:

- 1 pound pork stew meat, cut into strips
- 1 tablespoon Cajun seasoning
- 2 red bell peppers, sliced
- 14 ounces canned tomatoes, chopped
- 4 garlic cloves, minced
- 2 tablespoons coconut oil, melted
- A pinch of salt and black pepper

Directions:

Heat up a pan that fits the air fryer with the oil over medium-high heat, add the pork meat, seasoning, garlic, salt and pepper, toss and brown for 5 minutes. Add the remaining ingredients, toss, put the pan in the fryer and cook at 390 degrees F for 30 minutes. Divide everything between plates and serve.

Nutrition: calories 284, fat 13, fiber 4, carbs 6, protein 19

Roasted Spare Ribs

Prep time: 5 *minutes* | *Cooking time:* 45 *minutes* | *Servings:* 4

Ingredients:

- 2 tablespoons cocoa powder
- ½ teaspoon cinnamon powder
- ½ teaspoon chili powder
- 1 tablespoon coriander, chopped
- ½ teaspoon cumin, ground
- 2 racks of ribs
- A pinch of salt and black pepper
- Cooking spray

Directions:

Grease the ribs with the cooking spray, mix with the other ingredients and rub very well. Put the ribs in your air fryer's basket and cook at 390 degrees F for 45 minutes. Divide between plates and serve with a side salad.

Nutrition: calories 284, fat 14, fiber 5, carbs 7, protein 20

Cashew Pork Mix
Prep time: 5 minutes | Cooking time: 20 minutes | Servings: 4

Ingredients:

- 1 pound pork tenderloin, thinly cut into strips
- 1 egg, whisked
- 1 green onion, chopped
- 1 red bell pepper, sliced
- 1/3 cup cashews
- 1 tablespoon ginger, grated
- 3 garlic cloves, minced
- 1 tablespoon olive oil
- 2 tablespoons coconut aminos
- A pinch of salt and black pepper

Directions:

Heat up a pan that fits your air fryer with the oil over medium-high heat, add the pork and brown for 3 minutes. Add the rest of the ingredients except the egg, toss and cook for 1 minute more. Add the egg, toss, put the pan in the fryer and cook at 380 degrees F for 15 minutes, shaking the fryer halfway. Divide everything into bowls and serve.

Nutrition: calories 274, fat 12, fiber 4, carbs 6, protein 19

Pork and Ginger Sauce
Prep time: 5 minutes | Cooking time: 35 minutes | Servings: 4

Ingredients:

- 1 pound pork tenderloin, cut into strips
- 1 garlic clove, minced
- A pinch of salt and black pepper
- 1 tablespoon ginger, grated
- 3 tablespoons coconut aminos
- 2 tablespoons coconut oil, melted

Directions:

Heat up a pan that fits the air fryer with the oil over medium-high heat, add the meat and brown for 3 minutes. Add the rest of the ingredients, cook for 2 minutes more, put the pan in the fryer and cook at 380 degrees F for 30 minutes Divide between plates and serve with a side salad.

Nutrition: calories 284, fat 13, fiber 4, carbs 6, protein 18

Beef and Spinach Mix
Prep time: 5 minutes | Cooking time: 25 minutes | Servings: 4

Ingredients:

- 1 and ½ pounds beef meat, cubed
- Salt and black pepper to the taste
- 2 cup baby spinach
- 3 tablespoons olive oil
- 1 tablespoon sweet paprika
- ¼ cup beef stock

Directions:

In a pan that fits your air fryer mix all the ingredients except the spinach, toss, introduce the pan the fryer and cook at 390 degrees F for 20 minutes. Add the spinach, cook for 5 minutes more, divide everything between plates and serve.

Nutrition: calories 294, fat 13, fiber 3, carbs 6, protein 19

Beef Sauté
Prep time: 5 minutes | Cooking time: 25 minutes | Servings: 4

Ingredients:

- 1 pound beef meat, cut into thin strips
- 1 zucchini, roughly cubed
- 2 tablespoons coconut aminos
- 2 garlic cloves, minced
- ¼ cup cilantro, chopped
- 2 tablespoons avocado oil

Directions:

Heat up a pan that fits your air fryer with the oil over medium heat, add the meat and brown for 5 minutes. Add the rest of the ingredients, toss, put the pan in the fryer and cook at 380 degrees F for 20 minutes. Divide everything into bowls and serve.

Nutrition: calories 284, fat 13, fiber 4, carbs 6, protein 16

Beef Salad
Prep time: 5 minutes | Cooking time: 25 minutes | Servings: 4

Ingredients:

- 1 pound beef, cubed
- ¼ cup coconut aminos
- 1 tablespoon coconut oil, melted
- 6 ounces iceberg lettuce, shredded
- 2 tablespoons cilantro, chopped
- 2 tablespoons chives, chopped
- 1 zucchini, shredded
- ½ green cabbage head, shredded
- 2 tablespoons almonds, sliced
- 1 tablespoon sesame seeds
- ½ tablespoon white vinegar
- A pinch of salt and black pepper

Directions:
Heat up a pan that fits the air fryer with the oil over medium-high heat, add the meat and brown for 5 minutes. Add the aminos, zucchini, cabbage, salt and pepper, toss, put the pan in the fryer and cook at 370 degrees F for 20 minutes. Cool the mix down, transfer to a salad bowl, add the rest of the ingredients, toss well and serve.

Nutrition: calories 270, fat 12, fiber 4, carbs 6, protein 16

Coconut Beef and Broccoli Mix
Prep time: 5 minutes | Cooking time: 25 minutes | Servings: 4

Ingredients:

- 1 pound beef, cubed
- 1 broccoli head, florets separated
- 2 tablespoons olive oil
- 1 teaspoon coconut aminos
- 1 teaspoon stevia
- 1/3 cup balsamic vinegar
- 2 garlic cloves, minced

Directions:
In a pan that fits your air fryer, mix the beef with the rest of the ingredients, toss, put the pan in the fryer and cook at 390 degrees F for 225 minutes. Divide into bowls and serve hot.

Nutrition: calories 274, fat 12, fiber 4, carbs 6, protein 16

Creamy Beef
Prep time: 5 minutes | Cooking time: 25 minutes | Servings: 2

Ingredients:
- 1 pound beef, cut into strips
- 2 tablespoons coconut oil, melted
- A pinch of salt and black pepper
- 1 shallot, chopped
- 2 garlic cloves, minced
- 10 white mushrooms, sliced
- 1 tablespoon coconut aminos
- 1 tablespoon mustard
- 1 cup beef stock
- ¼ cup coconut cream
- ¼ cup parsley, chopped

Directions:
Heat up a pan that fits your air fryer with the oil over medium-high heat, add the meat and brown for 2 minutes. Add the garlic, shallots, mushrooms, salt and pepper, and cook for 3 minutes more. Add the remaining ingredients except the parsley, toss, put the pan in the fryer and cook at 390 degrees F for 20 minutes. Divide the mix into bowls and serve with parsley sprinkled on top.

Nutrition: calories 280, fat 134, fiber 5, carbs 7, protein 17

Beef and Radishes
Prep time: 5 minutes | Cooking time: 15 minutes | Servings: 2

Ingredients:
- 2 cups corned beef, cooked and shredded
- 2 garlic cloves, minced
- 1 pound radishes, quartered
- 2 spring onions, chopped
- A pinch of salt and black pepper

Directions:
In a pan that fits your air fryer, mix the beef with the rest of the ingredients, toss, put the pan in the fryer and cook at 390 degrees F for 15 minutes. Divide everything into bowls and serve.

Nutrition: calories 267, fat 13, fiber 2, carbs 5, protein 15

Beef and Fennel Pan
Prep time: 5 minutes | Cooking time: 20 minutes | Servings: 4

Ingredients:
- 2 tablespoons olive oil
- 1 pound beef, cut into strips
- 1 fennel bulb, sliced
- Salt and black pepper to the taste
- 1 teaspoon sweet paprika
- ¼ cup tomato sauce

Directions:
Heat up a pan that fits the air fryer with the oil over medium-high heat, add the beef and brown for 5 minutes. Add the rest of the ingredients, toss, put the pan in the machine and cook at 380 degrees F for 15 minutes. Divide the mix between plates and serve.

Nutrition: calories 284, fat 13, fiber 4, carbs 6, protein 15

Beef and Napa Cabbage Mix
Prep time: 5 minutes | Cooking time: 25 minutes | Servings: 4

Ingredients:
- 2 pounds beef, cubed
- ½ pound bacon, chopped
- 2 shallots, chopped
- 1 napa cabbage, shredded
- 2 garlic cloves, minced
- A pinch of salt and black pepper
- 2 tablespoons olive oil
- 1 teaspoon thyme, dried
- 1 cup beef stock

Directions:
Heat up a pan that fits the air fryer with the oil over medium-high heat, add the beef and brown for 3 minutes. Add the bacon, shallots and garlic and cook for 2 minutes more. Add the rest of the ingredients, toss, put the pan in the air fryer and cook at 390 degrees F for 20 minutes. Divide between plates and serve.

Nutrition: calories 284, fat 14, fiber 2, carbs 6, protein 19

Beef Meatloaf

Prep time: 5 minutes | Cooking time: 25 minutes | Servings: 4

Ingredients:
- 1 pound beef meat, ground
- 3 tablespoons almond meal
- Cooking spray
- 1 egg, whisked
- Salt and black pepper to the taste
- 1 tablespoon parsley, chopped
- 1 tablespoon oregano, chopped
- 1 yellow onion, chopped

Directions:
In a bowl, mix all the ingredients except the cooking spray, stir well and put in a loaf pan that fits the air fryer. Put the pan in the fryer and cook at 390 degrees F for 25 minutes. Slice and serve hot.

Nutrition: calories 284, fat 14, fiber 3, carbs 6, protein 18

Spicy Beef

Prep time: 5 minutes | Cooking time: 20 minutes | Servings: 4

Ingredients:
- 1 tablespoon hot paprika
- 4 beef steaks
- Salt and black pepper to the taste
- 1 tablespoon butter, melted

Directions:
In a bowl, mix the beef with the rest of the ingredients, rub well, transfer the steaks to your air fryer's basket and cook at 390 degrees F for 10 minutes on each side. Divide the steaks between plates and serve with a side salad.

Nutrition: calories 280, fat 12, fiber 4, carbs 6, protein 17

Ground Beef and Chilies
Prep time: 5 minutes | Cooking time: 20 minutes | Servings: 4

Ingredients:

- 1 pound beef, ground
- A pinch of salt and black pepper
- A drizzle of olive oil
- 2 spring onions, chopped
- 3 red chilies, chopped
- 1 cup beef stock
- 6 garlic cloves, minced
- 1 green bell pepper, chopped
- 8 ounces canned tomatoes, chopped
- 2 tablespoons chili powder

Directions:

Heat up a pan that fits your air fryer with the oil over medium-high heat, add the beef and brown for 3 minutes. Add the rest of the ingredients, toss, put the pan in the fryer and cook at 380 degrees F for 16 minutes. Divide into bowls and serve.

Nutrition: calories 276, fat 12, fiber 3, carbs 6, protein 17

Beef Steaks and Mushrooms
Prep time: 5 minutes | Cooking time: 25 minutes | Servings: 4

Ingredients:

- 4 beef steaks
- 1 tablespoon olive oil
- A pinch of salt and black pepper
- 2 tablespoons ghee, melted
- 2 garlic cloves, minced
- 5 cups wild mushrooms, sliced
- 1 tablespoon parsley, chopped

Directions:

Heat up a pan that fits the air fryer with the oil over medium-high heat, add the steaks and sear them for 2 minutes on each side. Add the rest of the ingredients, toss, transfer the pan to your air fryer and cook at 380 degrees F for 20 minutes. Divide between plates and serve.

Nutrition: calories 283, fat 14, fiber 4, carbs 6, protein 17

Roasted Rib Eye Steaks
Prep time: 5 minutes | Cooking time: 24 minutes | Servings: 4

Ingredients:
- 4 rib eye steaks
- A pinch of salt and black pepper
- 1 tablespoon olive oil
- 1 teaspoon sweet paprika
- 1 teaspoon cumin, ground
- 1 teaspoon rosemary, chopped

Directions:
In a bowl, mix the steaks with the rest of the ingredients, toss and put them in your air fryer's basket. Cook at 380 degrees F for 12 minutes on each side, divide between plates and serve.

Nutrition: calories 283, fat 12, fiber 3, carbs 6, protein 17

Adobo Beef
Prep time: 5 minutes | Cooking time: 30 minutes | Servings: 4

Ingredients:
- 1 pound beef roast, trimmed
- ½ teaspoon oregano, dried
- ¼ teaspoon garlic powder
- A pinch of salt and black pepper
- ½ teaspoon turmeric powder
- 1 tablespoon olive oil

Directions:
In a bowl, mix the roast with the rest of the ingredients, and rub well. Put the roast in the air fryer's basket and cook at 390 degrees F for 30 minutes. Slice the roast, divide it between plates and serve with a side salad.

Nutrition: calories 294, fat 12, fiber 3, carbs 6, protein 19

Beef Meatballs and Sauce

Prep time: 5 minutes | *Cooking time:* 25 minutes | *Servings:* 4

Ingredients:

- 2 tablespoons olive oil
- 2 spring onions, chopped
- 1 egg, whisked
- 2 tablespoons rosemary, chopped
- 2 pounds beef, ground
- 1 garlic clove, minced
- A pinch of salt and black pepper
- 24 ounces canned tomatoes, crushed

Directions:

In a bowl, mix the beef with all the ingredients except the oil and the tomatoes, stir well and shape medium meatballs out of this mix. Heat up a pan that fits the air fryer with the oil over medium-high heat, add the meatballs and cook for 2 minutes on each side. Add the tomatoes, toss, put the pan in the fryer and cook at 370 degrees F for 20 minutes. Divide into bowls and serve.

Nutrition: calories 273, fat 10, fiber 3, carbs 6, protein 15

Beef and Avocado Pan

Prep time: 5 minutes | *Cooking time:* 25 minutes | *Servings:* 4

Ingredients:

- 4 flank steaks
- 1 garlic clove, minced
- 1/3 cup beef stock
- 2 avocados, peeled, pitted and sliced
- 1 teaspoon chili flakes
- ½ cup basil, chopped
- 2 spring onions, chopped
- 2 teaspoons olive oil
- A pinch of salt and black pepper

Directions:

Heat up a pan that fits the air fryer with the oil over medium-high heat, add the steaks and cook for 2 minutes on each side. Add the rest of the ingredients except the avocados, put the pan in the air fryer and cook at 380 degrees F for 15 minutes. Add the avocado slices, cook for 5 minutes more, divide everything between plates and serve.

Nutrition: calories 273, fat 12, fiber 3, carbs 6, protein 18

Beef and Cheese Casserole
Prep time: 5 *minutes* | *Cooking time:* 30 *minutes* | *Servings:* 4

Ingredients:

- 1 tablespoon olive oil
- 1 and ½ cups coconut cream
- ½ cup parmesan, grated
- 1 pound beef, ground
- 1 bunch spring onions, chopped
- 1 tablespoons tomato sauce
- A pinch of salt and black pepper
- 2 cups cheddar cheese, ground
- 14 ounces canned tomatoes, chopped

Directions:

Heat up a pan with the oil over medium-high heat, add the beef and brown for 5 minutes. Add spring onions, tomatoes, salt and pepper and cook for 3-4 minutes more. Transfer this to a pan that fits the air fryer, pour the cream, sprinkle the parmesan and cheddar on top, put the pan in the fryer and cook at 380 degrees F for 20 minutes. Divide between plates and serve.

Nutrition: calories 273, fat 13, fiber 4, carbs 6, protein 18

Beef and Artichokes
Prep time: 5 *minutes* | *Cooking time:* 30 *minutes* | *Servings:* 4

Ingredients:

- 1 and ½ pounds beef stew meat, cubed
- A pinch of salt and black pepper
- 2 tablespoons olive oil
- 2 shallots, chopped
- 1 cup beef stock
- 2 garlic cloves, minced
- ½ teaspoon dill, chopped
- 12 ounces canned artichoke hearts, drained and chopped

Directions:

Heat up a pan that fits the air fryer with the oil over medium-high heat, add the meat and brown for 5 minutes. Add the rest of the ingredients except the dill, transfer the pan to your air fryer and cook at 380 degrees F for 25 minutes shaking the air fryer halfway. Divide everything into bowls and serve with the dill sprinkled on top.

Nutrition: calories 273, fat 13, fiber 4, carbs 6, protein 18

Mustard and Chives Beef
Prep time: 5 minutes | Cooking time: 20 minutes | Servings: 4

Ingredients:

- 3 garlic cloves, minced
- 1 and ½ pound beef, cut into strips
- 2 tablespoons coconut oil, melted
- 2 cups baby spinach
- 2 tablespoons chives, chopped
- 4 tablespoons mustard
- Salt and black pepper to the taste

Directions:

In a pan that fits the air fryer, combine all the ingredients, put the pan in the air fryer and cook at 390 degrees F for 20 minutes. Divide between plates and serve.

Nutrition: calories 283, fat 14, fiber 2, carbs 6, protein 19

Beef and Balsamic Marinade
Prep time: 5 minutes | Cooking time: 35 minutes | Servings: 4

Ingredients:

- 2 tablespoons olive oil
- 3 garlic cloves, minced
- Salt and black pepper to the taste
- 4 medium beef steaks
- 1 cup balsamic vinegar

Directions:

In a bowl, mix steaks with the rest of the ingredients, and toss. Transfer the steaks to your air fryer's basket and cook at 390 degrees F for 35 minutes, flipping them halfway. Divide between plates and serve with a side salad.

Nutrition: calories 273, fat 14, fiber 4, carbs 6, protein 19

Lamb Cakes
Prep time: 5 minutes | Cooking time: 30 minutes | Servings: 8

Ingredients:

- 2 spring onions, chopped
- 1 tablespoon garlic, minced
- 2 tablespoons cilantro, chopped
- 2 tablespoons mint, chopped
- A pinch of salt and black pepper
- Zest of 1 lemon
- Juice of 1 lemon
- ½ cup almond meal
- 3 eggs, whisked
- 2 and ½ pounds lamb meat, ground
- Cooking spray

Directions:

In a bowl, mix all the ingredients except the cooking spray, stir well and shape medium cakes out of this mix. Put the cakes in your air fryer, grease them with cooking spray and cook at 390 degrees F for 15 minutes on each side. Divide between plates and serve with a side salad.

Nutrition: calories 283, fat 13, fiber 4, carbs 6, protein 15

Roasted Lamb Chops
Prep time: 5 minutes | Cooking time: 24 minutes | Servings: 6

Ingredients:

- 12 lamb chops
- A pinch of salt and black pepper
- ½ cup cilantro, chopped
- 1 green chili pepper, chopped
- 1 garlic clove, minced
- Juice of 1 lime
- 3 tablespoons olive oil

Directions:

In a bowl, mix the lamb chops with the rest of the ingredients and rub well. Put the chops in your air fryer's basket and cook at 400 degrees F for 12 minutes on each side. Divide between plates and serve.

Nutrition: calories 284, fat 10, fiber 3, carbs 6, protein 16

Lamb Chops and Mint Sauce
Prep time: 5 minutes | Cooking time: 24 minutes | Servings: 4

Ingredients:
- 8 lamb chops
- A pinch of salt and black pepper
- 1 cup mint, chopped
- 1 garlic clove, minced
- Juice of 1 lemon
- 2 tablespoons olive oil

Directions:
In a blender, combine all the ingredients except the lamb and pulse well. Rub lamb chops with the mint sauce, put them in your air fryer's basket and cook at 400 degrees F for 12 minutes on each side. Divide everything between plates and serve.

Nutrition: calories 284, fat 14, fiber 3, carbs 6, protein 16

Lamb Skewers
Prep time: 10 minutes | Cooking time: 20 minutes | Servings: 4

Ingredients:
- 2 pounds lamb meat, cubed
- ¼ cup olive oil
- 1 tablespoon garlic, minced
- 1 tablespoon oregano, dried
- ½ teaspoon rosemary, dried
- 2 tablespoons lemon juice
- A pinch of salt and black pepper
- 1 tablespoon red vinegar
- 2 red bell peppers, cut into medium pieces

Directions:
In a bowl, mix all the ingredients and toss them well. Thread the lamb and bell peppers on skewers, place them in your air fryer's basket and cook at 380 degrees F for 10 minutes on each side. Divide between plates and serve with a side salad.

Nutrition: calories 274, fat 12, fiber 3, carbs 6, protein 16

Lamb with Olives and Tomatoes

Prep time: 5 minutes | Cooking time: 35 minutes | Servings: 4

Ingredients:

- 1 and ½ pounds lamb meat, cubed
- 2 tablespoons olive oil
- A pinch of salt and black pepper
- ¼ cup kalamata olives, pitted and sliced
- 4 garlic cloves, minced
- Zest of 1 lemon, grated
- 2 rosemary springs, chopped
- 6 tomatoes, cubed

Directions:

Heat up a pan that fits your air fryer with the oil over medium heat, add the meat and brown for 5 minutes. Add the rest of the ingredients, toss, put the pan in the air fryer and cook at 380 degrees F for 30 minutes. Divide everything into bowls and serve.

Nutrition: calories 274, fat 10, fiber 4, carbs 6, protein 15

Seasoned Lamb Mix

Prep time: 5 minutes | Cooking time: 35 minutes | Servings: 4

Ingredients:

- 1 pound lamb leg, boneless and sliced
- 2 tablespoons olive oil
- A pinch of salt and black pepper
- 2 garlic cloves, minced
- 1 tablespoon rosemary, chopped
- ½ cup walnuts, chopped
- ¼ teaspoon red pepper flakes
- ½ teaspoon mustard seeds
- ½ teaspoon Italian seasoning
- 1 tablespoon parsley, chopped

Directions:

In a bowl, mix the lamb with all the ingredients except the walnuts and parsley, rub well, put the slices your air fryer's basket and cook at 370 degrees F for 35 minutes, flipping the meat halfway. Divide between plates, sprinkle the parsley and walnuts on top and serve with a side salad.

Nutrition: calories 283, fat 13, fiber 4, carbs 6, protein 15

Chili Lamb and Cucumber Salsa

Prep time: 5 minutes | Cooking time: 35 minutes | Servings: 4

Ingredients:

- 1 tablespoon chipotle powder
- A pinch of salt and black pepper
- 1 and ½ pounds lamb loin, cubed
- 2 tablespoons red vinegar
- 4 tablespoons olive oil
- 2 tomatoes, cubed
- 2 cucumbers, sliced
- 2 spring onions, chopped
- Juice of ½ lemon
- ¼ cup mint, chopped

Directions:

Heat up a pan that fits your air fryer with half of the oil over medium-high heat, add the lamb, stir and brown for 5 minutes. Add the chipotle powder, salt pepper and the vinegar, toss, put the pan in the air fryer and cook at 380 degrees F for 30 minutes. In a bowl, mix tomatoes with cucumbers, onions, lemon juice, mint and the rest of the oil and toss. Divide the lamb between plates, top each serving with the cucumber salsa and serve.

Nutrition: calories 284, fat 13, fiber 3, carbs 6, protein 14

Lamb Curry

Prep time: 5 minutes | Cooking time: 35 minutes | Servings: 4

Ingredients:

- 2 tablespoons olive oil
- 1 and ½ pounds lamb meat, cubed
- A pinch of salt and black pepper
- 15 ounces canned tomatoes, chopped
- Juice of 2 limes
- 1 teaspoon sweet paprika
- 1 cup beef stock
- 1-inch ginger, grated
- 2 hot chilies, chopped
- 2 red bell peppers, chopped
- 4 garlic cloves, minced
- 2 teaspoons turmeric powder
- 1 tablespoon green curry paste

Directions:

Heat up a pan that fits your air fryer with the oil over medium heat, add the meat and brown for 5 minutes. Add the rest of the ingredients, toss, put the pan in the fryer and cook at 380 degrees F for 30 minutes. Divide everything into bowls and serve.

Nutrition: calories 284, fat 12, fiber 3, carbs 5, protein 16

Lamb Loin and Tomato Vinaigrette
Prep time: 10 minutes | Cooking time: 30 minutes | Servings: 4

Ingredients:
- 4 lamb loin slices
- A pinch of salt and black pepper
- 3 garlic cloves, minced
- 2 teaspoons thyme, chopped
- 2 tablespoons olive oil
- 1/3 cup parsley, chopped
- 1/3 cup sun-dried tomatoes, chopped
- 2 tablespoons balsamic vinegar
- 2 tablespoons water

Directions:
In a blender, combine all the ingredients except the lamb slices and pulse well. In a bowl, mix the lamb with the tomato vinaigrette and toss well. Put the lamb in your air fryer's basket and cook at 380 degrees F for 15 minutes on each side. Divide everything between plates and serve.

Nutrition: calories 273, fat 13, fiber 4, carbs 6, protein 17

Crusted Lamb Cutlets
Prep time: 5 minutes | Cooking time: 30 minutes | Servings: 4

Ingredients:
- 8 lamb cutlets
- A pinch of salt and black pepper
- 3 tablespoons mustard
- 3 tablespoons olive oil
- ½ cup coconut flakes
- ¼ cup parmesan, grated
- 2 tablespoons parsley, chopped
- 2 tablespoons chives, chopped
- 1 tablespoon rosemary, chopped

Directions:
In a bowl, mix the lamb cutlets with all the ingredients except the parmesan and the coconut flakes and toss well. Dredge the cutlets in parmesan and coconut flakes, put them in your air fryer's basket and cook at 390 degrees F for 15 minutes on each side. Divide between plates and serve.

Nutrition: calories 284, fat 13, fiber 3, carbs 6, protein 17

Lamb and Pine Nuts Meatballs
Prep time: 5 minutes | Cooking time: 30 minutes | Servings: 4

Ingredients:

- 1 and ½ pounds lamb, ground
- 1 scallion, chopped
- A pinch of salt and black pepper
- ½ cup pine nuts, toasted and chopped
- 1 tablespoon thyme, chopped
- 2 garlic cloves, minced
- 1 tablespoon olive oil
- 1 egg, whisked

Directions:

In a bowl, mix the lamb with the rest of the ingredients except the oil, stir well and shape medium meatballs out of this mix. Grease the meatballs with the oil, put them in your air fryer's basket and cook at 380 degrees F for 15 minutes on each side. Divide between plates and serve with a side salad.

Nutrition: calories 287, fat 12, fiber 3, carbs 6, protein 17.

Moroccan Lamb
Prep time: 5 minutes | Cooking time: 30 minutes| Servings: 4

Ingredients:

- 8 lamb cutlets
- A pinch of salt and black pepper
- 4 tablespoons olive oil
- ½ cup mint leaves
- 6 garlic cloves
- 1 tablespoon cumin, ground
- 1 tablespoon coriander seeds
- Zest of 2 lemons, grated
- 3 tablespoons lemon juice

Directions:

In a blender, combine all the ingredients except the lamb and pulse well. Rub the lamb cutlets with this mix, place them in your air fryer's basket and cook at 380 degrees F for 15 minutes on each side. Serve with a side salad.

Nutrition: calories 284, fat 13, fiber 3, carbs 5, protein 15

Rosemary Roasted Lamb Cutlets
Prep time: 5 minutes | Cooking time: 30 minutes | Servings: 4

Ingredients:
- 8 lamb cutlets
- 2 tablespoons olive oil
- A pinch of salt and black pepper
- 2 tablespoons rosemary, chopped
- 2 garlic cloves, minced
- A pinch of cayenne pepper

Directions:
In a bowl, mix the lamb with the rest of the ingredients and rub well. Put the lamb in the fryer's basket and cook at 380 degrees F for 30 minutes, flipping them halfway. Divide the cutlets between plates and serve.

Nutrition: calories 274, fat 12, fiber 3, carbs 5, protein 15

Herbed Lamb
Prep time: 10 minutes | Cooking time: 30 minutes | Servings: 4

Ingredients:
- 8 lamb cutlets
- A pinch of salt and black pepper
- A drizzle of olive oil
- 2 garlic cloves, minced
- ¼ cup mustard
- 1 tablespoon chives, chopped
- 1 tablespoon basil, chopped
- 1 tablespoon oregano, chopped
- 1 tablespoon mint chopped

Directions:
In a bowl, mix the lamb with the rest of the ingredients and rub well. Put the cutlets in your air fryer's basket and cook at 380 degrees F for 15 minutes on each side. Divide between plates and serve with a side salad.

Nutrition: calories 284, fat 13, fiber 3, carbs 6, protein 14

Smoked Lamb Chops
Prep time: 5 minutes | Cooking time: 20 minutes | Servings: 4

Ingredients:
- 4 lamb chops
- 4 garlic cloves, minced
- ½ teaspoon chili powder
- ¼ teaspoon smoked paprika
- 2 tablespoons olive oil
- A pinch of salt and black pepper

Directions:
In a bowl, mix the lamb with the rest of the ingredients and toss well. Transfer the chops to your air fryer's basket and cook at 390 degrees F for 10 minutes on each side. Serve with a side salad.

Nutrition: calories 274, fat 12, fiber 4, carbs 6, protein 17

Lamb Chops and Marjoram Sauce
Prep time: 5 minutes | Cooking time: 25 minutes | Servings: 4

Ingredients:
- 4 lamb chops
- 2 tablespoons olive oil
- Salt and black pepper to the taste
- 1 tablespoon marjoram, chopped
- 3 garlic cloves, minced
- 1 teaspoon thyme, dried
- ½ cup tomato sauce

Directions:
Heat up a pan that fits the air fryer with the oil over medium-high heat, add the lamb chops and brown for 5 minutes. Add the rest of the ingredients, toss, put the pan in the fryer and cook at 390 degrees F for 20 minutes more. Divide into bowls and serve right away.

Nutrition: calories 274, fat 14, fiber 3, carbs 6, protein 14

Lamb and Creamy Cilantro Sauce
Prep time: 5 minutes | Cooking time: 30 minutes | Servings: 4

Ingredients:
- 1 pound lamb, cubed
- 1 cup coconut cream
- 3 tablespoons sweet paprika
- 2 tablespoons olive oil
- 2 tablespoons cilantro, chopped
- Salt and black pepper to the taste

Directions:
Heat up a pan that fits your air fryer with the oil over medium-high heat, add the meat and brown for 5 minutes. Add the rest of the ingredients, toss, put the pan in the air fryer and cook at 380 degrees F for 25 minutes. Divide everything into bowls and serve.

Nutrition: calories 287, fat 13, fiber 2, carbs 6, protein 12

Greek Lamb Chops
Prep time: 5 minutes | Cooking time: 30 minutes | Servings: 4

Ingredients:
- 4 lamb chops
- A pinch of salt and black pepper
- 1 cup Greek yogurt
- 2 tablespoons coconut oil, melted
- 1 teaspoon lemon zest, grated
- ½ teaspoon turmeric powder

Directions:
In a bowl, mix the lamb chops with the rest of the ingredients and toss well. Put the chops in your air fryer's basket and cook at 380 degrees F for 15 minutes on each side. Divide between plates and serve.

Nutrition: calories 283, fat 13, fiber 3, carbs 6, protein 15

Lamb Ribs and Rhubarb
Prep time: 5 minutes | Cooking time: 30 minutes | Servings: 4

Ingredients:

- 1 and ½ pound lamb ribs
- A pinch of salt and black pepper
- 1 tablespoon black peppercorns, ground
- 1 tablespoon white peppercorns, ground
- 1 tablespoon fennel seeds, ground
- 1 tablespoon coriander seeds, ground
- 4 rhubarb stalks, chopped
- ¼ cup balsamic vinegar
- 2 tablespoons olive oil

Directions:

Heat up a pan that fits your air fryer with the oil over medium heat, add the lamb and brown for 2 minutes. Add the rest of the ingredients, toss, bring to a simmer for 2 minutes and take off the heat. Put the pan in the fryer and cook at 380 degrees for 25 minutes. Divide everything into bowls and serve.

Nutrition: calories 283, fat 13, fiber 2, carbs 6, protein 17

Lamb Meatloaf
Prep time: 5 minutes | Cooking time: 35 minutes | Servings: 4

Ingredients:

- 2 pounds lamb, ground
- A pinch of salt and black pepper
- ½ teaspoon hot paprika
- A drizzle of olive oil
- 2 tablespoons parsley, chopped
- 2 tablespoons cilantro, chopped
- 1 teaspoon cumin, ground
- ¼ teaspoon cinnamon powder
- 1 teaspoon coriander, ground
- 1 egg
- 2 tablespoons tomato sauce
- 4 scallions, chopped
- 1 teaspoon lemon juice

Directions:

In a bowl, combine the lamb with the rest of the ingredients except the oil and stir really well. Grease a loaf pan that fits the air fryer with the oil, add the lamb mix and shape the meatloaf. Put the pan in the air fryer and cook at 380 degrees F for 35 minutes. Slice and serve.

Nutrition: calories 263, fat 12, fiber 3, carbs 6, protein 15

Ketogenic Air Fryer Vegetable Recipes

Italian Asparagus Mix
Prep time: 5 *minutes* | *Cooking time:* 10 *minutes* | *Servings:* 4

Ingredients:

- 1 pound asparagus, trimmed
- 2 tablespoons olive oil
- A pinch of salt and black pepper
- 2 cups mozzarella, shredded
- ½ cup balsamic vinegar
- 2 cups cherry tomatoes, halved

Directions:

In a pan that fits your air fryer, mix the asparagus with the rest of the ingredients except the mozzarella and toss. Put the pan in the air fryer and cook at 400 degrees F for 10 minutes. Divide between plates and serve.

Nutrition: calories 200, fat 6, fiber 2, carbs 3, protein 6

Roasted Asparagus
Prep time: 5 *minutes* | *Cooking time:* 10 *minutes* | *Servings:* 4

Ingredients:

- 1 pound asparagus, trimmed
- 3 tablespoons olive oil
- A pinch of salt and black pepper
- 1 tablespoon sweet paprika

Directions:

In a bowl, mix the asparagus with the rest of the ingredients and toss. Put the asparagus in your air fryer's basket and cook at 400 degrees F for 10 minutes. Divide between plates and serve.

Nutrition: calories 200, fat 5, fiber 2, carbs 4, protein 6

Asparagus and Yogurt Sauce
Prep time: 4 minutes | Cooking time: 10 minutes | Servings: 4

Ingredients:
- 1 pound asparagus, trimmed
- 2 tablespoons olive oil
- A pinch of salt and black pepper
- 1 teaspoon garlic powder
- 1 teaspoon oregano, dried
- 1 cup Greek yogurt
- 1 cup basil, chopped
- ½ cup parsley, chopped
- ¼ cup chives, chopped
- ¼ cup lemon juice
- 2 garlic cloves, minced

Directions:
In a bowl, mix the asparagus with the oil, salt, pepper, oregano and garlic powder, and toss. Put the asparagus in the air fryer's basket and cook at 400 degrees F for 10 minutes. Meanwhile, in a blender, mix the yogurt with basil, chives, parsley, lemon juice and garlic cloves and pulse well. Divide the asparagus between plates, drizzle the sauce all over and serve.

Nutrition: calories 194, fat 6, fiber 2, carbs 4, protein 8

Asparagus and Tomatoes
Prep time: 5 minutes | Cooking time: 10 minutes | Servings: 4

Ingredients:
- 1 pound asparagus, trimmed
- 2 cups cherry tomatoes, halved
- ¼ cup parmesan, grated
- ½ cup balsamic vinegar
- 2 tablespoons olive oil
- A pinch of salt and black pepper

Directions:
In a bowl, mix the asparagus with the rest of the ingredients except the parmesan, and toss. Put the asparagus and tomatoes in your air fryer's basket and cook at 400 degrees F for 10 minutes Divide between plates and serve with the parmesan sprinkled on top.

Nutrition: calories 173, fat 4, fiber 2, carbs 4, protein 8

Bacon Asparagus Mix
Prep time: 5 minutes | Cooking time: 10 minutes | Servings: 4

Ingredients:

- 2 pounds asparagus, trimmed
- 2 tablespoons olive oil
- 1 cup cheddar cheese, shredded
- 4 garlic cloves, minced
- 4 bacon slices, cooked and crumbled

Directions:

In a bowl, mix the asparagus with the other ingredients except the bacon, toss and put in your air fryer's basket. Cook at 400 degrees F for 10 minutes, divide between plates, sprinkle the bacon on top and serve.

Nutrition: calories 172, fat 6, fiber 2, carbs 5, protein 8

Mustard Asparagus Mix
Prep time: 5 minutes | Cooking time: 12 minutes | Servings: 4

Ingredients:

- 1 pound asparagus, trimmed
- 2 tablespoons olive oil
- ¼ cup mustard
- 3 garlic cloves, minced
- ½ cup parmesan, grated

Directions:

In a bowl, mix the asparagus with the oil, garlic and mustard and toss really well. Put the asparagus spears in your air fryer's basket and cook at 400 degrees F for 12 minutes. Divide between plates, sprinkle the parmesan on top and serve.

Nutrition: calories 162, fat 4, fiber 4, carbs 6, protein 9

Lemon Asparagus
Prep time: 5 minutes | Cooking time: 12 minutes | Servings: 4

Ingredients:
- 1 pound asparagus, trimmed
- A pinch of salt and black pepper
- 2 tablespoons olive oil
- 3 garlic cloves, minced
- 3 tablespoons parmesan, grated
- Juice of 1 lemon

Directions:
In a bowl, mix the asparagus with the rest of the ingredients and toss. Put the asparagus in your air fryer's basket and cook at 390 degrees F for 12 minutes. Divide between plates and serve.

Nutrition: calories 175, fat 5, fiber 2, carbs 4, protein 8

Broccoli Casserole
Prep time: 5 minutes | Cooking time: 30 minutes | Servings: 4

Ingredients:
- 3 tablespoons ghee, melted
- 15 ounces coconut cream
- 2 eggs, whisked
- 2 cups cheddar, grated
- 1 cup parmesan, grated
- 1 tablespoon mustard
- 1 pound broccoli florets
- A pinch of salt and black pepper
- 1 tablespoon parsley, chopped

Directions:
Grease a baking pan that fits the air fryer with the ghee and arrange the broccoli on the bottom. Add the cream, mustard, salt, pepper and the eggs and toss. Sprinkle the cheese on top, put the pan in the air fryer and cook at 380 degrees F for 30 minutes. Divide between plates and serve.

Nutrition: calories 244, fat 12, fiber 3, carbs 5, protein 12

Vinegar Broccoli Mix

Prep time: 5 minutes | Cooking time: 25 minutes | Servings: 4

Ingredients:

- 1 broccoli head, florets separated
- 2 shallots, chopped
- A pinch of salt and black pepper
- ½ cup cranberries
- ½ cup almonds, chopped
- 6 bacon slices, cooked and crumbled
- 3 tablespoons balsamic vinegar

Directions:

In a pan that fits the air fryer, combine the broccoli with the rest of the ingredients and toss. Put the pan in the air fryer and cook at 380 degrees F for 25 minutes. Divide between plates and serve.

Nutrition: calories 173, fat 7, fiber 2, carbs 4, protein 8

Broccoli and Tomato Sauce

Prep time: 5 minutes | Cooking time: 15 minutes | Servings: 4

Ingredients:

- 1 broccoli head, florets separated
- Salt and black pepper to the taste
- ½ cup tomato sauce
- 1 tablespoon sweet paprika
- ¼ cup scallions, chopped
- 1 tablespoon olive oil

Directions:

In a pan that fits the air fryer, combine the broccoli with the rest of the ingredients, toss, put the pan in the fryer and cook at 380 degrees F for 15 minutes. Divide between plates and serve.

Nutrition: calories 163, fat 5, fiber 2, carbs 4, protein 8

Chili Broccoli

Prep time: 5 minutes | *Cooking time:* 15 minutes | *Servings:* 4

Ingredients:

- 1 pound broccoli florets
- 2 tablespoons olive oil
- 2 tablespoons chili sauce
- Juice of 1 lime
- A pinch of salt and black pepper

Directions:

In a bowl, mix the broccoli with the other ingredients and toss well. Put the broccoli in your air fryer's basket and cook at 400 degrees F for 15 minutes. Divide between plates and serve.

Nutrition: calories 173, fat 6, fiber 2, carbs 6, protein 8

Parmesan Broccoli and Asparagus

Prep time: 5 minutes | *Cooking time:* 15 minutes | *Servings:* 4

Ingredients:

- 1 broccoli head, florets separated
- ½ pound asparagus, trimmed
- Juice of 1 lime
- Salt and black pepper to the taste
- 2 tablespoons olive oil
- 3 tablespoons parmesan, grated

Directions:

In a bowl, mix the asparagus with the broccoli and all the other ingredients except the parmesan, toss, transfer to your air fryer's basket and cook at 400 degrees F for 15 minutes. Divide between plates, sprinkle the parmesan on top and serve.

Nutrition: calories 172, fat 5, fiber 2, carbs 4, protein 9

Broccoli and Almonds
Prep time: 5 minutes | Cooking time: 12 minutes | Servings: 4

Ingredients:
- 1 pound broccoli florets
- 3 garlic cloves, minced
- A pinch of salt and black pepper
- 3 tablespoons coconut oil, melted
- ½ cup almonds, chopped
- 1 tablespoon chives, chopped
- 2 tablespoons red vinegar

Directions:
In a bowl, mix the broccoli with the garlic, salt, pepper, vinegar and the oil and toss. Put the broccoli in your air fryer's basket and cook at 380 degrees F for 12 minutes. Divide between plates and serve with almonds and chives sprinkled on top.

Nutrition: calories 180, fat 4, fiber 2, carbs 4, protein 6

Butter Broccoli Mix
Prep time: 5 minutes | Cooking time: 15 minutes | Servings: 4

Ingredients:
- 1 pound broccoli florets
- A pinch of salt and black pepper
- 1 teaspoons sweet paprika
- ½ tablespoon butter, melted

Directions:
In a bowl, mix the broccoli with the rest of the ingredients, and toss. Put the broccoli in your air fryer's basket, cook at 350 degrees F for 15 minutes, divide between plates and serve.

Nutrition: calories 130, fat 3, fiber 3, carbs 4, protein 8

Kale and Bell Peppers Mix
Prep time: 5 minutes | Cooking time: 10 minutes | Servings: 4

Ingredients:
- 2 cups kale, torn
- A pinch of salt and black pepper
- 1 and ½ cups avocado, peeled, pitted and cubed
- 1 cup red bell pepper, sliced
- ¼ cup olive oil
- 1 tablespoon mustard
- 2 tablespoons lime juice
- 1 tablespoon white vinegar

Directions:
In a pan that fits the air fryer, combine the kale with salt, pepper, avocado and half of the oil, toss, put in your air fryer and cook at 360 degrees F for 10 minutes. In a bowl, combine the kale mix with the rest of the ingredients, toss and serve.

Nutrition: calories 131, fat 3, fiber 2, carbs 4, protein 5

Balsamic Kale
Prep time: 2 minutes | Cooking time: 12 minutes | Servings: 6

Ingredients:
- 2 tablespoons olive oil
- 3 garlic cloves, minced
- 2 and ½ pounds kale leaves
- Salt and black pepper to the taste
- 2 tablespoons balsamic vinegar

Directions:
In a pan that fits the air fryer, combine all the ingredients and toss. Put the pan in your air fryer and cook at 300 degrees F for 12 minutes. Divide between plates and serve.

Nutrition: calories 122, fat 4, fiber 3, carbs 4, protein 5

Creamy Kale

Prep time: 5 minutes | Cooking time: 15 minutes | Servings: 4

Ingredients:

- 2 pounds kale, torn
- A pinch of salt and black pepper
- 2 tablespoons olive oil
- 2 garlic cloves, minced
- 1 and ½ cups coconut cream
- ½ teaspoon nutmeg, ground
- ½ cup parmesan, grated

Directions:

In a pan that fits your air fryer, mix the kale with the rest of the ingredients, toss, introduce the pan in the fryer and cook at 400 degrees F for 15 minutes. Divide between plates and serve.

Nutrition: calories 135, fat 3, fiber 2, carbs 4, protein 6

Kale and Olives

Prep time: 5 minutes | Cooking time: 15 minutes | Servings: 4

Ingredients:

- 1 an ½ pounds kale, torn
- 2 tablespoons olive oil
- Salt and black pepper to the taste
- 1 tablespoon hot paprika
- 2 tablespoons black olives, pitted and sliced

Directions:

In a pan that fits the air fryer, combine all the ingredients and toss. Put the pan in your air fryer, cook at 370 degrees F for 15 minutes, divide between plates and serve.

Nutrition: calories 154, fat 3, fiber 2, carbs 4, protein 6

Kale and Mushrooms Mix
Prep time: 5 minutes | Cooking time: 15 minutes | Servings: 4

Ingredients:
- 1 pound brown mushrooms, sliced
- 1 pound kale, torn
- Salt and black pepper to the taste
- 2 tablespoons olive oil
- 14 ounces coconut milk

Directions:
In a pan that fits your air fryer, mix the kale with the rest of the ingredients and toss. Put the pan in the fryer, cook at 380 degrees F for 15 minutes, divide between plates and serve.

Nutrition: calories 162, fat 4, fiber 1, carbs 3, protein 5

Oregano Kale
Prep time: 5 minutes | Cooking time: 10 minutes | Servings: 4

Ingredients:
- 1 pound kale, torn
- 1 tablespoon olive oil
- A pinch of salt and black pepper
- 2 tablespoons oregano, chopped

Directions:
In a pan that fits the air fryer, combine all the ingredients and toss. Put the pan in the air fryer and cook at 380 degrees F for 10 minutes. Divide between plates and serve.

Nutrition: calories 140, fat 3, fiber 2, carbs 3, protein 5

Kale and Brussels Sprouts
Prep time: 5 minutes | Cooking time: 15 minutes | Servings: 8

Ingredients:
- 1 pound Brussels sprouts, trimmed
- 2 cups kale, torn
- 1 tablespoon olive oil
- Salt and black pepper to the taste
- 3 ounces mozzarella, shredded

Directions:

In a pan that fits the air fryer, combine all the ingredients except the mozzarella and toss. Put the pan in the air fryer and cook at 380 degrees F for 15 minutes. Divide between plates, sprinkle the cheese on top and serve.

Nutrition: calories 170, fat 5, fiber 3, carbs 4, protein 7

Italian Olives Mix
Prep time: 5 minutes | Cooking time: 15 minutes | Servings: 4

Ingredients:
- 2 cups black olives, pitted and halved
- A handful basil, chopped
- 2 rosemary springs, chopped
- 2 red bell peppers, sliced
- 12 ounces tomatoes, chopped
- 4 garlic cloves, minced
- 2 tablespoons olive oil

Directions:

In a pan that fits the air fryer, combine the olives with the rest of the ingredients, toss, put the pan in the fryer and cook at 380 degrees F for 15 minutes. Divide between plates and serve.

Nutrition: calories 173, fat 6, fiber 2, carbs 4, protein 5

Olives and Zucchini

Prep time: 5 minutes | Cooking time: 12 minutes | Servings: 4

Ingredients:

- 4 zucchinis, sliced
- 1 cup kalamata olives, pitted
- Salt and black pepper to the taste
- 2 tablespoons lime juice
- 2 tablespoons olive oil
- 2 teaspoons balsamic vinegar

Directions:

In a pan that fits your air fryer, mix the olives with all the other ingredients, toss, introduce in the fryer and cook at 390 degrees F for 12 minutes. Divide the mix between plates and serve.

Nutrition: calories 150, fat 4, fiber 2, carbs 4, protein 5

Artichokes and Olives

Prep time: 5 minutes | Cooking time: 15 minutes | Servings: 4

Ingredients:

- 14 ounces canned artichoke hearts, drained
- 1 tablespoon olive oil
- 2 cups black olives, pitted
- 3 garlic cloves, minced
- ½ cup tomato sauce
- 1 teaspoon garlic powder

Directions:

In a pan that fits your air fryer, mix the olives with the artichokes and the other ingredients, toss, put the pan in the fryer and cook at 350 degrees F for 15 minutes. Divide the mix between plates and serve.

Nutrition: calories 180, fat 4, fiber 3, carbs 5, protein 6

Spicy Olives and Avocado Mix
Prep time: 5 minutes | Cooking time: 15 minutes | Servings: 4

Ingredients:

- 2 cups kalamata olives, pitted
- 2 small avocados, pitted, peeled and sliced
- ¼ cup cherry tomatoes, halved
- Juice of 1 lime
- 1 tablespoon coconut oil, melted

Directions:

In a pan that fits the air fryer, combine the olives with the other ingredients, toss, put the pan in your air fryer and cook at 370 degrees F for 15 minutes. Divide the mix between plates and serve.

Nutrition: calories 153, fat 3, fiber 3, carbs 4, protein 6

Olives, Green beans and Bacon
Prep time: 5 minutes | Cooking time: 15 minutes | Servings: 4

Ingredients:

- ½ pound green beans, trimmed and halved
- 1 cup black olives, pitted and halved
- ¼ cup bacon, cooked and crumbled
- 1 tablespoon olive oil
- ¼ cup tomato sauce

Directions:

In a pan that fits the air fryer, combine all the ingredients, toss, put the pan in the air fryer and cook at 380 degrees F for 15 minutes. Divide between plates and serve.

Nutrition: calories 160, fat 4, fiber 3, carbs 5, protein 4

Cajun Olives and Peppers
Prep time: 4 minutes | Cooking time: 12 minutes | Servings: 4

Ingredients:
- 1 tablespoon olive oil
- ½ pound mixed bell peppers, sliced
- 1 cup black olives, pitted and halved
- ½ tablespoon Cajun seasoning

Directions:
In a pan that fits the air fryer, combine all the ingredients. Put the pan it in your air fryer and cook at 390 degrees F for 12 minutes. Divide the mix between plates and serve.

Nutrition: calories 151, fat 3, fiber 2, carbs 4, protein 5

Olives and Cilantro Vinaigrette
Prep time: 5 minutes | Cooking time: 12 minutes | Servings: 4

Ingredients:
- 2 tablespoons balsamic vinegar
- A bunch of cilantro, chopped
- Salt and black pepper to the taste
- 1 tablespoon olive oil
- 2 cups black olives, pitted
- 1 cup baby spinach

Directions:
In a pan that fits the air fryer, combine all the ingredients and toss. Put the pan in the air fryer and cook at 370 degrees F for 12 minutes. Transfer to bowls and serve.

Nutrition: calories 132, fat 4, fiber 2, carbs 4, protein 4

Celery and Brussels Sprouts
Prep time: 5 minutes | Cooking time: 12 minutes | Servings: 4

Ingredients:

- 1 celery stalks, roughly chopped
- 1 cup coconut cream
- Salt and black pepper to the taste
- 1 tablespoon parsley, chopped
- 1 tablespoon coconut oil, melted
- ½ pound Brussels sprouts, halved

Directions:

Heat up a pan that fits the air fryer with the oil over medium heat, add the sprouts and celery, stir and cook for 2 minutes. Add the cream and the remaining ingredients, toss, put the pan in the air fryer and cook at 380 degrees F for 10 minutes. Transfer to bowls and serve.

Nutrition: calories 140, fat 3, fiber 2, carbs 5, protein 6

Lemon Bell Peppers Mix
Prep time: 5 minutes | Cooking time: 15 minutes | Servings: 4

Ingredients:

- 1 and ½ pounds mixed bell peppers, halved and deseeded
- 2 teaspoons lemon zest, grated
- 2 tablespoons balsamic vinegar
- 2 tablespoons lemon juice
- A handful parsley, chopped
- A drizzle of olive oil

Directions:

Put the peppers in your air fryer's basket and cook at 350 degrees F for 15 minutes. Peel the bell peppers, mix them with the rest of the ingredients, toss and serve.

Nutrition: calories 151, fat 2, fiber 3, carbs 5, protein 5

Tomato, Avocado and Green Beans
Prep time: 5 minutes | Cooking time: 15 minutes | Servings: 4

Ingredients:
- 1 pint mixed cherry tomatoes, halved
- 1 avocado, peeled, pitted and cubed
- ¼ pound green beans, trimmed and halved
- 2 tablespoons olive oil

Directions:
In a pan that fits your air fryer, mix the tomatoes with the rest of the ingredients, toss, put the pan in the machine and cook at 360 degrees F for 15 minutes. Transfer to bowls and serve.

Nutrition: calories 151, fat 3, fiber 2, carbs 4, protein 4

Tomato and Asparagus
Prep time: 5 minutes | Cooking time: 15 minutes | Servings: 4

Ingredients:
- 1 pound asparagus, trimmed
- 2 green onions, chopped
- 1 jalapeno pepper, chopped
- 1 tablespoon olive oil
- 2 teaspoons chili powder
- A pinch of salt and black pepper
- 10 cherry tomatoes, halved

Directions:
In a pan that fits your air fryer, mix the asparagus with tomatoes and the rest of the ingredients, toss, put the pan in the fryer and cook at 390 degrees F for 15 minutes. Divide the mix between plates and serve.

Nutrition: calories 173, fat 4, fiber 2, carbs 4, protein 6

Tomato and Kale Salad
Prep time: 5 minutes | Cooking time: 15 minutes | Servings: 4

Ingredients:
- 10 cherry tomatoes, halved
- ½ pound kale leaves, torn
- Salt and black pepper to the taste
- ¼ cup veggie stock
- 2 tablespoons tomato sauce

Directions:

In a pan that fits your air fryer, mix tomatoes with the remaining ingredients, toss, put the pan in the fryer and cook at 360 degrees F for 15 minutes. Divide between plates and serve right away.

Nutrition: calories 161, fat 2, fiber 2, carbs 4, protein 6

Garlic Tomatoes Mix
Prep time: 5 minutes | Cooking time: 15 minutes | Servings: 4

Ingredients:
- 1 tablespoon olive oil
- 1 pound cherry tomatoes, halved
- 1 tablespoon dill, chopped
- 6 garlic cloves, minced
- 1 tablespoon balsamic vinegar
- Salt and black pepper to the taste

Directions:

In a pan that fits the air fryer, combine all the ingredients, toss gently, put the pan in the air fryer and cook at 380 degrees F for 15 minutes. Divide between plates and serve.

Nutrition: calories 121, fat 3, fiber 2, carbs 4, protein 6

Broccoli and Tomatoes Mix
Prep time: 5 minutes | Cooking time: 15 minutes | Servings: 4

Ingredients:

- 1 broccoli head, florets separated
- 2 cups cherry tomatoes, quartered
- A pinch of salt and black pepper
- 1 tablespoon cilantro, chopped
- Juice of 1 lime
- A drizzle of olive oil

Directions:

In a pan that fits the air fryer, combine the broccoli with tomatoes and the rest of the ingredients except the cilantro, toss, put the pan in the air fryer and cook at 380 degrees F for 15 minutes. Divide between plates and serve with cilantro sprinkled on top.

Nutrition: calories 141, fat 3, fiber 2, carbs 4, protein 5

Dill and Garlic Green Beans
Prep time: 5 minutes | Cooking time: 15 minutes | Servings: 4

Ingredients:

- 1 pound green beans, trimmed
- 1 tablespoon coconut oil, melted
- 2 garlic cloves, minced
- Salt and black pepper to the taste
- ½ cup bacon, cooked and chopped
- 2 tablespoons dill, chopped

Directions:

In a pan that fits the air fryer, combine the green beans with the rest of the ingredients, toss, put the pan in the machine and cook at 390 degrees F for 15 minutes. Divide everything between plates and serve.

Nutrition: calories 180, fat 3, fiber 2, carbs 4, protein 6

Green Beans and Lime Sauce
Prep time: 5 minutes | Cooking time: 8 minutes | Servings: 4

Ingredients:
- 1 pound green beans, trimmed
- 1 tablespoon lime juice
- A pinch of salt and black pepper
- 2 tablespoons ghee, melted
- 1 teaspoon chili powder

Directions:
In a bowl, mix the ghee with the rest of the ingredients except the green beans and whisk really well. Mix the green beans with the lime sauce, toss, put them in your air fryer's basket and cook at 400 degrees F for 8 minutes. Serve right away.

Nutrition: calories 151, fat 4, fiber 2, carbs 4, protein 6

Savoy Cabbage Mix
Prep time: 5 minutes | Cooking time: 15 minutes | Servings: 4

Ingredients:
- 1 Savoy cabbage head, shredded
- Salt and black pepper to the taste
- 1 and ½ tablespoons ghee, melted
- ¼ cup coconut cream
- 1 tablespoon dill, chopped

Directions:
In a pan that fits the air fryer, combine all the ingredients except the coconut cream, toss, put the pan in the air fryer and cook at 390 degrees F for 10 minutes. Add the cream, toss, cook for 5 minutes more, divide between plates and serve.

Nutrition: calories 173, fat 5, fiber 3, carbs 5, protein 8

Savoy Cabbage and Tomatoes Mix
Prep time: 5 minutes | Cooking time: 15 minutes | Servings: 4

Ingredients:
- 1 savoy cabbage, shredded
- 2 spring onions, chopped
- 2 tablespoons tomato sauce
- Salt and black pepper to the taste
- 1 tablespoon parsley, chopped

Directions:
In a pan that fits your air fryer, mix the cabbage the rest of the ingredients except the parsley, toss, put the pan in the fryer and cook at 360 degrees F for 15 minutes. Divide between plates and serve with parsley sprinkled on top.

Nutrition: calories 163, fat 4, fiber 3, carbs 6, protein 7

Turmeric Cabbage Mix
Prep time: 5 minutes | Cooking time: 15 minutes | Servings: 4

Ingredients:
- 1 green cabbage head, shredded
- ¼ cup ghee, melted
- 2 teaspoons turmeric powder
- 1 tablespoon dill, chopped

Directions:
In a pan that fits your air fryer, mix the cabbage with the rest of the ingredients except the dill, toss, put the pan in the fryer and cook at 370 degrees F for 15 minutes. Divide everything between plates and serve with dill sprinkled on top.

Nutrition: calories 173, fat 5, fiber 3, carbs 6, protein 7

Lemon Endives
Prep time: 5 minutes | Cooking time: 15 minutes | Servings: 4

Ingredients:
- 3 tablespoons ghee, melted
- 12 endives, trimmed
- A pinch of salt and black pepper
- 1 tablespoon lemon juice

Directions:
In a bowl, mix the endives with the ghee, salt, pepper and lemon juice and toss. Put the endives in the fryer's basket and cook at 350 degrees F for 15 minutes. Divide between plates and serve.

Nutrition: calories 163, fat 4, fiber 3, carbs 5, protein 6

Balsamic Endives
Prep time: 5 minutes | Cooking time: 15 minutes | Servings: 4

Ingredients:
- 4 endives, halved
- 1 tablespoon olive oil
- A pinch of salt and black pepper
- 2 tablespoons balsamic vinegar
- 3 tablespoons ghee, melted
- 3 tablespoons oregano, chopped

Directions:
Heat up a pan that fits your air fryer with the oil and the ghee over medium heat, add the rest of the ingredients except the endives, whisk and cook for 3 minutes. Add the endives, toss and take off the heat. Put the endives in your air fryer's basket and cook at 350 degrees F for 12 minutes. Divide between plates and serve with the ghee mix drizzled on top.

Nutrition: calories 143, fat 4, fiber 3, carbs 6, protein 7

Endives and Walnuts Mix
Prep time: 5 minutes | Cooking time: 15 minutes | Servings: 4

Ingredients:
- 4 endives, trimmed
- 3 tablespoons olive oil
- A pinch of salt and black pepper
- 1 teaspoon mustard
- 2 tablespoons white vinegar
- ½ cup walnuts, chopped

Directions:
In a bowl, mix the oil with salt, pepper, mustard and vinegar and whisk really well. Add the endives, toss and transfer them to your air fryer's basket. Cook at 350 degrees F for 15 minutes, divide between plates and serve with walnuts sprinkled on top.

Nutrition: calories 154, fat 4, fiber 3, carbs 6, protein 7

Cheesy Endives
Prep time: 5 minutes | Cooking time: 15 minutes | Servings: 4

Ingredients:
- 4 endives, trimmed
- A pinch of salt and black pepper
- ¼ cup goat cheese, crumbled
- 1 teaspoon lemon zest, grated
- 1 tablespoon lemon juice
- 2 tablespoons chives, chopped
- 2 tablespoons olive oil

Directions:
In a bowl, mix the endives with the other ingredients except the cheese and chives and toss well. Put the endives in your air fryer's basket and cook at 380 degrees F for 15 minutes. Divide the corn between plates and serve with cheese and chives sprinkled on top.

Nutrition: calories 140, fat 4, fiber 3, carbs 5, protein 7

Endives and Mushrooms Sauté
Prep time: 5 minutes | *Cooking time:* 15 minutes | *Servings:* 4

Ingredients:

- 4 endives, trimmed and sliced
- A pinch of salt and black pepper
- 1 tablespoon olive oil
- 2 shallots, chopped
- 1 cup white mushrooms, sliced
- ½ cup parmesan, grated
- 1 tablespoon parsley, chopped
- Juice of ½ lemon

Directions:

Heat up a pan that fits the air fryer with the oil over medium-high heat, add the shallots and sauté for 2 minutes. Add the mushrooms, stir and cook for 1-2 minutes more. Add the rest of the ingredients except the parmesan and the parsley, toss, put the pan in the air fryer and cook at 380 degrees F for 10 minutes. Divide everything between plates and serve.

Nutrition: calories 170, fat 4, fiber 3, carbs 5, protein 8

Asparagus and Fennel
Prep time: 5 minutes | *Cooking time:* 15 minutes | *Servings:* 4

Ingredients:

- 1 pound asparagus, trimmed
- 1 fennel bulb, quartered
- A pinch of salt and black pepper
- 2 cherry tomatoes, chopped
- 2 chili peppers, chopped
- 2 tablespoons cilantro, chopped
- 2 tablespoons parsley, chopped
- 2 tablespoons olive oil
- 2 tablespoons lemon juice

Directions:

Heat up a pan that fits the air fryer with the oil over medium-high heat, add chili peppers and the fennel and sauté for 2 minutes. Add the rest of the ingredients, toss, put the pan in the air fryer and cook at 380 degrees F for 12 minutes. Divide everything between plates and serve.

Nutrition: calories 163, fat 4, fiber 2, carbs 4, protein 7

Fennel and Collard Greens Sauté
Prep time: 5 minutes | Cooking time: 12 minutes | Servings: 4

Ingredients:

- 1 pound collard greens, trimmed
- 2 fennel bulbs, trimmed and quartered
- 2 tablespoons olive oil
- Salt and black pepper to the taste
- ½ cup tomato sauce

Directions:

In a pan that fits your air fryer, mix the collard greens with the fennel and the rest of the ingredients, toss, put the pan in the fryer and cook at 350 degrees F for 12 minutes. Divide everything between plates and serve.

Nutrition: calories 163, fat 4, fiber 3, carbs 5, protein 6

Mustard Greens and Green Beans
Prep time: 10 minutes | Cooking time: 12 minutes | Servings: 4

Ingredients:

- 1 bunch mustard greens, trimmed
- 1 pound green beans, halved
- 2 tablespoons olive oil
- ¼ cup tomato puree
- 3 garlic cloves, minced
- Salt and black pepper to the taste
- 1 tablespoon balsamic vinegar

Directions:

In a pan that fits your air fryer, mix the mustard greens with the rest of the ingredients, toss, put the pan in the fryer and cook at 350 degrees F for 12 minutes. Divide everything between plates and serve.

Nutrition: calories 163, fat 4, fiber 3, carbs 4, protein 7

Fennel and Blueberry Mix
Prep time: 5 minutes | Cooking time: 12 minutes | Servings: 4

Ingredients:

- 2 fennel bulbs, trimmed and sliced
- 1 cup blueberries
- 2 ounces mozzarella, shredded
- 2 tablespoons mint, chopped
- A pinch of salt and black pepper

- 2 tablespoons olive oil
- 1 and ½ teaspoons mustard
- 1 teaspoon coconut aminos
- 1 teaspoon balsamic vinegar
- 2 tablespoons shallots, chopped

Directions:

Heat up a pan that fits the air fryer with the oil over medium heat, add the shallots, stir and cook for 2 minutes. Add the fennel and the blueberries, toss gently and take the pan off the heat. In a bowl, combine the mint with mustard, coconut aminos and vinegar and whisk well. Add this over the fennel mix, toss, put the pan in the air fryer and cook at 350 degrees F for 10 minutes. Divide between plates and serve with the mozzarella sprinkled on top.

Nutrition: calories 162, fat 5, fiber 3, carbs 4, protein 6

Nutmeg Endives Mix
Prep time: 5 minutes | Cooking time: 10 minutes | Servings: 4

Ingredients:

- 4 endives, trimmed and halved
- Salt and black pepper to the taste
- 1 tablespoon coconut oil, melted

- 1 tablespoon lemon juice
- ½ teaspoon nutmeg, ground
- 1 tablespoon chives, chopped

Directions:

In a bowl, mix the endives with the rest of the ingredients except the chives and toss well. Put the endives in your air fryer's basket and cook at 360 degrees F for 10 minutes. Divide the endives between plates, sprinkle the chives on top and serve.

Nutrition: calories 162, fat 4, fiber 3, carbs 5, protein 7

Ketogenic Air Fryer Dessert Recipes

Almond Cupcakes
Prep time: 5 minutes | *Cooking time:* 25 minutes | *Servings:* 4

Ingredients:

- 1/3 cup coconut flour
- ½ cup cocoa powder
- 3 tablespoons stevia
- ½ teaspoon baking soda
- 1 teaspoon baking powder
- 4 eggs, whisked
- 1 teaspoon vanilla extract
- 4 tablespoons coconut oil, melted
- ¼ cup almond milk
- Cooking spray

Directions:

In a bowl, mix all the ingredients except the cooking spray and whisk well. Grease a cupcake tin that fits the air fryer with the cooking spray, pour the cupcake mix, put the pan in your air fryer, cook at 350 degrees F for 25 minutes, cool down and serve.

Nutrition: calories 103, fat 4, fiber 2, carbs 6, protein 3

Coconut Cookies
Prep time: 5 minutes | *Cooking time:* 15 minutes | *Servings:* 8

Ingredients:

- 1 and ½ cups coconut, shredded
- 2 tablespoons erythritol
- ½ teaspoon baking powder
- ¼ teaspoon almond extract
- 2 eggs, whisked

Directions:

In a bowl, mix all the ingredients and whisk well. Scoop 8 servings of this mix on a baking sheet that fits the air fryer which you've lined with parchment paper. Put the baking sheet in your air fryer and cook at 350 degrees F for 15 minutes. Serve cold.

Nutrition: calories 125, fat 7, fiber 1, carbs 5, protein 4

Coconut Bars

Prep time: 5 minutes | Cooking time: 40 minutes | Servings: 12

Ingredients:

- 1 and ¼ cups almond flour
- 1 cup swerve
- 1 cup butter, melted
- ½ cup coconut cream
- 1 and ½ cups coconut, flaked
- 1 egg yolk
- ¾ cup walnuts, chopped
- ½ teaspoon vanilla extract

Directions:

In a bowl, mix the flour with half of the swerve and half of the butter, stir well and press this on the bottom of a baking pan that fits the air fryer. Introduce this in the air fryer and cook at 350 degrees F for 15 minutes. Meanwhile, heat up a pan with the rest of the butter over medium heat, add the remaining swerve and the rest of the ingredients, whisk, cook for 1-2 minutes, take off the heat and cool down. Spread this well over the crust, put the pan in the air fryer again and cook at 350 degrees F for 25 minutes. Cool down, cut into bars and serve.

Nutrition: calories 182, fat 12, fiber 2, carbs 4, protein 4

Lemon Bars

Prep time: 10 minutes | Cooking time: 35 minutes | Servings: 8

Ingredients:

- ½ cup butter, melted
- 3 tablespoons erythritol
- 1 and ¾ cups almond flour
- 3 eggs, whisked
- Zest of 1 lemon, grated
- Juice of 3 lemons

Directions:

In a bowl, mix 1 cup flour with half of the erythritol and the butter, stir well and press into a baking dish that fits the air fryer lined with parchment paper. Put the dish in your air fryer and cook at 350 degrees F for 10 minutes. Meanwhile, in a bowl, mix the rest of the flour with the remaining erythritol and the other ingredients and whisk well. Spread this over the crust, put the dish in the air fryer once more and cook at 350 degrees F for 25 minutes. Cool down, cut into bars and serve.

Nutrition: calories 210, fat 12, fiber 1, carbs 4, protein 8

Sweet Zucchini Bread
Prep time: 10 minutes | Cooking time: 40 minutes | Servings: 12

Ingredients:
- 2 cups almond flour
- 2 teaspoons baking powder
- ¾ cup swerve
- ½ cup coconut oil, melted
- 1 teaspoon lemon juice
- 1 teaspoon vanilla extract
- 3 eggs, whisked
- 1 cup zucchini, shredded
- 1 tablespoon lemon zest
- Cooking spray

Directions:
In a bowl, mix all the ingredients except the cooking spray and stir well. Grease a loaf pan that fits the air fryer with the cooking spray, line with parchment paper and pour the loaf mix inside. Put the pan in the air fryer and cook at 330 degrees F for 40 minutes. Cool down, slice and serve.

Nutrition: calories 143, fat 11, fiber 1, carbs 3, protein 3

Lemon Coconut Pie
Prep time: 10 minutes | Cooking time: 35 minutes | Servings: 8

Ingredients:
- 2 eggs, whisked
- ¾ cup swerve
- ¼ cup coconut flour
- 2 tablespoons butter, melted
- 1 teaspoon lemon zest, grated
- 1 teaspoon baking powder
- 1 teaspoon vanilla extract
- ½ teaspoon lemon extract
- 4 ounces coconut, shredded
- Cooking spray

Directions:
In a bowl, combine all the ingredients except the cooking spray and stir well. Grease a pie pan that fits the air fryer with the cooking spray, pour the mixture inside, put the pan in the air fryer and cook at 360 degrees F for 35 minutes. Slice and serve warm.

Nutrition: calories 212, fat 15, fiber 2, carbs 6, protein 4

Strawberry Tart
Prep time: 5 minutes | Cooking time: 20 minutes | Servings: 8

Ingredients:
- 5 egg whites
- 1/3 cup swerve
- 1 and ½ cups almond flour
- Zest of 1 lemon, grated
- 1 teaspoon baking powder
- 1 teaspoon vanilla extract
- 1/3 cup butter, melted
- 2 cups strawberries, sliced
- Cooking spray

Directions:
In a bowl, whisk egg whites well. Add the rest of the ingredients except the cooking spray gradually and whisk everything. Grease a tart pan with the cooking spray, and pour the strawberries mix. Put the pan in the air fryer and cook at 370 degrees F for 20 minutes. Cool down, slice and serve.

Nutrition: calories 182, fat 12, fiber 1, carbs 6, protein 5

Coconut Donuts
Prep time: 5 minutes | Cooking time: 15 minutes | Servings: 4

Ingredients:
- 8 ounces coconut flour
- 2 tablespoons stevia
- 1 egg, whisked
- 2 and ½ tablespoons butter, melted
- 4 ounces coconut milk
- 1 teaspoon baking powder

Directions:
In a bowl, mix all the ingredients and whisk well. Shape donuts from this mix, place them in your air fryer's basket and cook at 370 degrees F for 15 minutes. Serve warm.

Nutrition: calories 190, fat 12, fiber 1, carbs 4, protein 6

Butter Cookies
Prep time: 10 minutes | *Cooking time:* 20 minutes | *Servings:* 12

Ingredients:
- 2 eggs, whisked
- 1 tablespoon heavy cream
- ½ cup butter, melted
- 2 teaspoons vanilla extract
- 2 and ¾ cup almond flour
- Cooking spray
- ¼ cup swerve

Directions:

In a bowl, mix all the ingredients except the cooking spray and stir well. Shape 12 balls out of this mix, put them on a baking sheet that fits the air fryer greased with cooking spray and flatten them. Put the baking sheet in the air fryer and cook at 350 degrees F for 20 minutes. Serve the cookies cold.

Nutrition: calories 234, fat 13, fiber 2, carbs 4, protein 7

Ginger Cookies
Prep time: 10 minutes | *Cooking time:* 15 minutes | *Servings:* 12

Ingredients:
- 2 cups almond flour
- 3 tablespoons swerve
- ¼ cup butter, melted
- 1 egg
- 2 teaspoons ginger, grated
- 1 teaspoon vanilla extract
- ¼ teaspoon nutmeg, ground
- ¼ teaspoon cinnamon powder

Directions:

In a bowl, mix all the ingredients and whisk well. Spoon small balls out of this mix on a lined baking sheet that fits the air fryer lined with parchment paper and flatten them. Put the sheet in the fryer and cook at 360 degrees F for 15 minutes. Cool the cookies down and serve.

Nutrition: calories 220, fat 13, fiber 2, carbs 4, protein 3

Raspberry Muffins
Prep time: 10 minutes | Cooking time: 20 minutes | Servings: 8

Ingredients:
- ¾ cup raspberries
- ¼ cup ghee, melted
- 1 egg
- ¼ cup swerve
- ¼ cup coconut flour
- 2 tablespoons almond meal
- 1 teaspoon cinnamon powder
- 3 tablespoons cream cheese
- ½ teaspoon baking soda
- ½ teaspoon baking powder
- Cooking spray

Directions:
In a bowl, mix all the ingredients except the cooking spray and whisk well. Grease a muffin pan that fits the air fryer with the cooking spray, pour the raspberry mix, put the pan in the machine and cook at 350 degrees F for 20 minutes. Serve the muffins cold.

Nutrition: calories 223, fat 7, fiber 2, carbs 4, protein 5

Strawberry Jam
Prep time: 10 minutes | Cooking time: 20 minutes | Servings: 12

Ingredients:
- ¼ cup swerve
- 8 ounces strawberries, sliced
- 1 tablespoon lemon juice
- ¼ cup water

Directions:
In a pan that fits the air fryer, combine all the ingredients, put the pan in the machine and cook at 380 degrees F for 20 minutes. Divide the mix into cups, cool down and serve.

Nutrition: calories 100, fat 1, fiber 0, carbs 1, protein 1

Blueberry Cream
Prep time: 4 *minutes* | *Cooking time:* 20 *minutes* | *Servings:* 6

Ingredients:
- 2 cups blueberries
- Juice of ½ lemon
- 2 tablespoons water
- 1 teaspoon vanilla extract
- 2 tablespoons swerve

Directions:
In a bowl, mix all the ingredients and whisk well. Divide this into 6 ramekins, put them in the air fryer and cook at 340 degrees F for 20 minutes Cool down and serve.

Nutrition: calories 123, fat 2, fiber 2, carbs 4, protein 3

Cocoa Cake
Prep time: 5 *minutes* | *Cooking time:* 20 *minutes* | *Servings:* 8

Ingredients:
- 2 egg
- 3 tablespoons swerve
- 3 tablespoons coconut oil, melted
- ¼ cup coconut milk
- 4 tablespoons almond flour
- 1 tablespoon cocoa powder
- ½ teaspoon baking powder

Directions:
In a bowl, mix all the ingredients and stir well. Pour this into a cake pan that fits the air fryer, put the pan in the machine and cook at 340 degrees F for 20 minutes. Slice and serve.

Nutrition: calories 191, fat 12, fiber 2, carbs 4, protein 6

Blackberry Chia Jam

Prep time: 10 minutes | Cooking time: 30 minutes | Servings: 12

Ingredients:

- 3 cups blackberries
- ¼ cup swerve
- 4 tablespoons lemon juice
- 4 tablespoons chia seeds

Directions:

In a pan that fits the air fryer, combine all the ingredients and toss. Put the pan in the machine and cook at 300 degrees F for 30 minutes. Divide into cups and serve cold.

Nutrition: calories 100, fat 2, fiber 1, carbs 3, protein 1

Mixed Berries Cream

Prep time: 5 minutes | Cooking time: 30 minutes | Servings: 6

Ingredients:

- 12 ounces blackberries
- 6 ounces raspberries
- 12 ounces blueberries
- ¼ cup swerve
- 2 ounces coconut cream

Directions:

In a bowl, mix all the ingredients and whisk well. Divide this into 6 ramekins, put them in your air fryer and cook at 320 degrees F for 30 minutes. Cool down and serve it.

Nutrition: calories 100, fat 1, fiber 1, carbs 2, protein 2

Cream Cheese Brownies
Prep time: 10 minutes | Cooking time: 25 minutes | Servings: 6

Ingredients:

- 6 tablespoons cream cheese, soft
- 3 eggs, whisked
- 2 tablespoons cocoa powder
- 3 tablespoons coconut oil, melted
- ¼ cup almond flour
- ¼ cup coconut flour
- ¼ teaspoon baking soda
- 1 teaspoon vanilla extract
- ½ cup almond milk
- 3 tablespoons swerve
- Cooking spray

Directions:

Grease a cake pan that fits the air fryer with the cooking spray. In a bowl, mix rest of the ingredients, whisk well and pour into the pan. Put the pan in your air fryer, cook at 370 degrees F for 25 minutes, cool the brownies down, slice and serve.

Nutrition: calories 182, fat 12, fiber 2, carbs 4, protein 6

Avocado Brownies
Prep time: 10 minutes | Cooking time: 30 minutes | Servings: 12

Ingredients:

- 1 cup avocado, peeled and mashed
- ½ teaspoon vanilla extract
- 4 tablespoons cocoa powder
- 3 tablespoons coconut oil, melted
- 2 eggs, whisked
- ½ cup dark chocolate, unsweetened and melted
- ¾ cup almond flour
- 1 teaspoon baking powder
- ¼ teaspoon baking soda
- 1 teaspoon stevia

Directions:

In a bowl, mix the flour with stevia, baking powder and soda and stir. Add the rest of the ingredients gradually, whisk and pour into a cake pan that fits the air fryer after you lined it with parchment paper. Put the pan in your air fryer and cook at 350 degrees F for 30 minutes. Cut into squares and serve cold.

Nutrition: calories 155, fat 6, fiber 2, carbs 6, protein 4

Cream and Coconut Cups
Prep time: 5 minutes | Cooking time: 10 minutes | Servings: 6

Ingredients:
- 2 tablespoons butter, melted
- 8 ounces cream cheese, soft
- 3 tablespoons coconut, shredded and unsweetened
- 3 eggs
- 4 tablespoons swerve

Directions:
In a bowl, mix all the ingredients and whisk really well. Divide into small ramekins, put them in the fryer and cook at 320 degrees F and bake for 10 minutes. Serve cold.

Nutrition: calories 164, fat 4, fiber 2, carbs 5, protein 5

Cream Cheese and Zucchinis Bars
Prep time: 10 minutes | Cooking time: 15 minutes | Servings: 12

Ingredients:
- 3 tablespoons coconut oil, melted
- 6 eggs
- 3 ounces zucchini, shredded
- 2 teaspoons vanilla extract
- ½ teaspoon baking powder
- 4 ounces cream cheese
- 2 tablespoons erythritol

Directions:
In a bowl, combine all the ingredients and whisk well. pour this into a baking dish that fits your air fryer lined with parchment paper, introduce in the fryer and cook at 320 degrees F, bake for 15 minutes. Slice and serve cold.

Nutrition: calories 178, fat 8, fiber 3, carbs 4, protein 5

Walnut and Vanilla Bars
Prep time: 5 minutes | Cooking time: 16 minutes | Servings: 4

Ingredients:
- 1 egg
- 1/3 cup cocoa powder
- 3 tablespoons swerve
- 7 tablespoons ghee, melted
- 1 teaspoon vanilla extract
- ¼ cup almond flour
- ¼ cup walnuts, chopped
- ½ teaspoon baking soda

Directions:
In a bowl, mix all the ingredients and stir well. Spread this on a baking sheet that fits your air fryer lined with parchment paper, put it in the fryer and cook at 330 degrees F and bake for 16 minutes. Leave the bars to cool down, cut and serve.

Nutrition: calories 182, fat 12, fiber 1, carbs 3, protein 6

Blackberry and Chocolate Cream
Prep time: 5 minutes | Cooking time: 15 minutes | Servings: 6

Ingredients:
- 1 cup blackberries
- 2 eggs
- ½ cup heavy cream
- ½ cup ghee, melted
- ¼ cup chocolate, melted
- 1 tablespoon stevia
- 2 teaspoons baking powder

Directions:
In a bowl, mix the blackberries with the rest of the ingredients, whisk well, divide into ramekins, put them in the fryer and cook at 340 degrees F for 15 minutes. Serve cold.

Nutrition: calories 150, fat 2, fiber 2, carbs 4, protein 7

Almond Butter Cookies
Prep time: 5 minutes | Cooking time: 12 minutes | Servings: 12

Ingredients:
- 1 teaspoon vanilla extract
- 1 cup almond butter, soft
- 1 egg
- 2 tablespoons erythritol

Directions:

In a bowl, mix all the ingredients and whisk well. Spread this on a cookie sheet that fits the air fryer lined with parchment paper, introduce in the fryer and cook at 350 degrees F and bake for 12 minutes. Cool down and serve.

Nutrition: calories 130, fat 12, fiber 1, carbs 3, protein 5

Yogurt Cake
Prep time: 5 minutes | Cooking time: 30 minutes | Servings: 12

Ingredients:
- 6 eggs, whisked
- 1 teaspoon vanilla extract
- 1 teaspoon baking powder
- 9 ounces coconut flour
- 4 tablespoons stevia
- 8 ounces Greek yogurt

Directions:

In a bowl, mix all the ingredients and whisk well. Pour this into a cake pan that fits the air fryer lined with parchment paper, put the pan in the air fryer and cook at 330 degrees F for 30 minutes.

Nutrition: calories 181, fat 13, fiber 2, carbs 4, protein 5

Chocolate Pudding
Prep time: 10 minutes | Cooking time: 20 minutes | Servings: 6

Ingredients:
- 24 ounces cream cheese, soft
- 2 tablespoons almond meal
- ¼ cup erythritol
- 3 eggs, whisked
- 1 tablespoon vanilla extract
- ½ cup heavy cream
- 12 ounces dark chocolate, melted

Directions:

In a bowl mix all the ingredients and whisk well. Divide this into 6 ramekins, put them in your air fryer and cook at 320 degrees F for 20 minutes. Keep in the fridge for 1 hour before serving.

Nutrition: calories 200, fat 7, fiber 2, carbs 4, protein 6

Plum Cake
Prep time: 10 minutes | *Cooking time:* 30 minutes | *Servings:* 8

Ingredients:
- ½ cup butter, soft
- 3 eggs
- ½ cup swerve
- ¼ teaspoon almond extract
- 1 tablespoon vanilla extract
- 1 and ½ cups almond flour
- ½ cup coconut flour
- 2 teaspoons baking powder
- ¾ cup almond milk
- 4 plums, pitted and chopped

Directions:

In a bowl, mix all the ingredients and whisk well. Pour this into a cake pan that fits the air fryer after you've lined it with parchment paper, put the pan in the machine and cook at 370 degrees F for 30 minutes. Cool the cake down, slice and serve.

Nutrition: calories 183, fat 4, fiber 3, carbs 4, protein 7

Baked Plums
Prep time: 5 minutes | *Cooking time:* 20 minutes | *Servings:* 6

Ingredients:
- 6 plums, cut into wedges
- 1 teaspoon ginger, ground
- ½ teaspoon cinnamon powder
- Zest of 1 lemon, grated
- 2 tablespoons water
- 10 drops stevia

Directions:

In a pan that fits the air fryer, combine the plums with the rest of the ingredients, toss gently, put the pan in the air fryer and cook at 360 degrees F for 20 minutes. Serve cold.

Nutrition: calories 170, fat 5, fiber 1, carbs 3, protein 5

Plum Cream
Prep time: 5 minutes | *Cooking time:* 20 minutes | *Servings:* 4

Ingredients:
- 1 pound plums, pitted and chopped
- ¼ cup swerve
- 1 tablespoon lemon juice
- 1 and ½ cups heavy cream

Directions:

In a bowl, mix all the ingredients and whisk well. Divide this into 4 ramekins, put them in the air fryer and cook at 340 degrees F for 20 minutes. Serve cold.

Nutrition: calories 171, fat 4, fiber 2, carbs 4, protein 4

Lemon Blackberries Cake
Prep time: 10 minutes | Cooking time: 25 minutes | Servings: 4

Ingredients:
- 2 eggs, whisked
- 4 tablespoons swerve
- 2 tablespoons ghee, melted
- ¼ cup almond milk
- 1 and ½ cups almond flour
- 1 cup blackberries, chopped
- ½ teaspoon baking powder
- 1 teaspoon lemon zest, grated
- 1 teaspoon lemon juice

Directions:

In a bowl, mix all the ingredients and whisk well. Pour this into a cake pan that fits the air fryer lined with parchment paper, put the pan in your air fryer and cook at 340 degrees F for 25 minutes. Cool the cake down, slice and serve.

Nutrition: calories 193, fat 5, fiber 1, carbs 4, protein 4

Cinnamon Plums
Prep time: 5 minutes | Cooking time: 20 minutes | Servings: 4

Ingredients:
- 2 teaspoons cinnamon powder
- 4 plums, halved
- 4 tablespoons butter, melted
- 3 tablespoons swerve

Directions:

In a pan that fits your air fryer, mix the plums with the rest of the ingredients, toss, put the pan in the air fryer and cook at 300 degrees F for 20 minutes. Divide into cups and serve cold.

Nutrition: calories 162, fat 3, fiber 2, carbs 4, protein 5

Strawberries Stew
Prep time: 10 minutes | Cooking time: 20 minutes | Servings: 4

Ingredients:
- 1 pound strawberries, halved
- 4 tablespoons stevia
- 1 tablespoon lemon juice
- 1 and ½ cups water

Directions:

In a pan that fits your air fryer, mix all the ingredients, toss, put it in the fryer and cook at 340 degrees F for 20 minutes. Divide the stew into cups and serve cold.

Nutrition: calories 176, fat 2, fiber 1, carbs 3, protein 5

Blueberries and Chocolate Cream

Prep time: 5 minutes | *Cooking time:* 20 minutes | *Servings:* 4

Ingredients:

- 2 cups blueberries
- 3 tablespoons chocolate, melted
- 4 tablespoons erythritol
- 3 tablespoons cream cheese, soft

Directions:

In a pan that fits the air fryer, combine all the ingredients, whisk, put the pan in the fryer and cook at 340 degrees F for 20 minutes. Divide into bowls and serve cold.

Nutrition: calories 200, fat 6, fiber 2, carbs 4, protein 5

Cocoa and Nuts Bombs

Prep time: 5 minutes | *Cooking time:* 8 minutes | *Servings:* 12

Ingredients:

- 2 cups macadamia nuts, chopped
- 4 tablespoons coconut oil, melted
- 1 teaspoon vanilla extract
- ¼ cup cocoa powder
- 1/3 cup swerve

Directions:

In a bowl, mix all the ingredients and whisk well. Shape medium balls out of this mix, place them in your air fryer and cook at 300 degrees F for 8 minutes. Serve cold.

Nutrition: calories 120, fat 12, fiber 1, carbs 2, protein 1

Avocado and Raspberries Cake

Prep time: 10 minutes | *Cooking time:* 30 minutes | *Servings:* 4

Ingredients:

- 4 ounces raspberries
- 2 avocados, peeled, pitted and mashed
- 1 cup almond flour
- 3 teaspoons baking powder
- 3 tablespoons swerve
- 4 tablespoons butter, melted
- 4 eggs, whisked

Directions:

In a bowl, mix all the ingredients, toss, pour this into a cake pan that fits the air fryer after you've lined it with parchment paper, put the pan in the fryer and cook at 340 degrees F for 30 minutes. Leave the cake to cool down, slice and serve.

Nutrition: calories 193, fat 4, fiber 2, carbs 5, protein 5

Spiced Avocado Pudding
Prep time: 5 *minutes* | *Cooking time:* 25 *minutes* | *Serving:* 6

Ingredients:

- 4 small avocados, peeled, pitted and mashed
- 2 eggs, whisked
- 1 cup coconut milk
- ¾ cup swerve
- 1 teaspoon cinnamon powder
- ½ teaspoon ginger powder

Directions:

In a bowl, mix all the ingredients and whisk well. Pour into a pudding mould, put it in the air fryer and cook at 350 degrees F for 25 minutes. Serve warm.

Nutrition: calories 192, fat 8, fiber 2, carbs 5, protein 4

Lime Berry Pudding
Prep time: 5 *minutes* | *Cooking time:* 15 *minutes* | *Servings:* 6

Ingredients:

- 2 cups coconut cream
- 1/3 cup blackberries
- 1/3 cup blueberries
- 3 tablespoons swerve
- Zest of 1 lime, grated

Directions:

In a blender, combine all the ingredients and pulse well. Divide this into 6 small ramekins, put them in your air fryer and cook at 340 degrees F for 15 minutes. Serve cold.

Nutrition: calories 173, fat 3, fiber 1, carbs 4, protein 4

Strawberry Cake
Prep time: 10 *minutes* | *Cooking time:* 35 *minutes* | *Servings:* 6

Ingredients:

- 1 pound strawberries, chopped
- 1 cup cream cheese, soft
- ¼ cup swerve
- 1 tablespoon lime juice
- 1 egg, whisked
- 1 teaspoon vanilla extract
- 3 tablespoons coconut oil, melted
- 1 cup almond flour
- 2 teaspoons baking powder

Directions:

In a bowl, mix all the ingredients, stir well and pour this into a cake pan lined with parchment paper. Put the pan in the air fryer, cook at 350 degrees F for 35 minutes, cool down, slice and serve.

Nutrition: calories 200, fat 6, fiber 2, carbs 4, protein 6

Coconut and Avocado Cake
Prep time: 5 minutes | Cooking time: 40 minutes | Servings: 6

Ingredients:
- 2 tablespoons ghee, melted
- 1 cup coconut , shredded
- 1 cup mashed avocado
- 3 tablespoons stevia
- 1 teaspoon cinnamon powder
- 2 teaspoons cinnamon powder

Directions:

In a bowl, mix all the ingredients and stir well. Pour this into a cake pan lined with parchment paper, place the pan in the fryer and cook at 340 degrees F for 40 minutes. Cool the cake down, slice and serve.

Nutrition: calories 192, fat 4, fiber 2, carbs 5, protein 7

Creamy Chia Seeds Pudding
Prep time: 10 minutes | Cooking time: 25 minutes | Servings: 6

Ingredients:
- 2 cups coconut cream
- 6 egg yolks, whisked
- 2 tablespoons stevia
- ¼ cup chia seeds
- 2 teaspoons cinnamon powder
- 1 tablespoon ghee, melted

Directions:

In a bowl, mix all the ingredients, whisk, divide into 6 ramekins, place them all in your air fryer and cook at 340 degrees F for 25 minutes. Cool the puddings down and serve.

Nutrition: calories 180, fat 4, fiber 2 carbs 5, protein 7

Cauliflower Rice and Plum Pudding
Prep time: 5 minutes | Cooking time: 25 minutes | Servings: 4

Ingredients:
- 1 and ½ cups cauliflower rice
- 2 cups coconut milk
- 3 tablespoons stevia
- 2 tablespoons ghee, melted
- 4 plums, pitted and roughly chopped

Directions:

In a bowl, mix all the ingredients, toss, divide into ramekins, put them in the air fryer, and cook at 340 degrees F for 25 minutes. Cool down and serve.

Nutrition: calories 221, fat 4, fiber 1, carbs 3, protein 3

Avocado Granola

Prep time: 4 minutes | Cooking time: 8 minutes | Servings: 6

Ingredients:
- 1 cup avocado, peeled, pitted and cubed
- ½ cup coconut flakes
- 2 tablespoons ghee, melted
- ¼ cup walnuts, chopped
- ¼ cup almonds, chopped
- 2 tablespoons stevia

Directions:

In a pan that fits your air fryer, mix all the ingredients, toss, put the pan in the fryer and cook at 320 degrees F for 8 minutes. Divide into bowls and serve right away.

Nutrition: calories 170, fat 3, fiber 2, carbs 4, protein 3

Currant Cream

Prep time: 5 minutes | Cooking time: 30 minutes | Servings: 4

Ingredients:
- 7 cups red currants
- ¼ cup swerve
- 1 cup water
- 6 sage leaves

Directions:

In a pan that fits your air fryer, mix all the ingredients, toss, put the pan in the fryer and cook at 330 degrees F for 30 minutes. Discard sage leaves, divide into cups and serve cold.

Nutrition: calories 171, fat 4, fiber 2, carbs 3, protein 6

Currant Pudding

Prep time: 5 minutes | Cooking time: 20 minutes | Servings: 6

Ingredients:
- 1 cup red currants, blended
- 1 cup black currants, blended
- 3 tablespoons stevia
- 1 cup coconut cream

Directions:

In a bowl, combine all the ingredients and stir well. Divide into ramekins, put them in the fryer and cook at 340 degrees F for 20 minutes. Serve the pudding cold.

Nutrition: calories 200, fat 4, fiber 2, carbs 4, protein 6

Currant Cookies

Prep time: 5 minutes | Cooking time: 30 minutes | Servings: 6

Ingredients:

- 2 cups almond flour
- 2 teaspoons baking soda
- ½ cup ghee, melted
- ½ cup swerve
- 1 teaspoon vanilla extract
- ½ cup currants

Directions:

In a bowl, mix all the ingredients and whisk well. Spread this on a baking sheet lined with parchment paper, put the pan in the air fryer and cook at 350 degrees F for 30 minutes. Cool down, cut into rectangles and serve.

Nutrition: calories 172, fat 5, fiber 2, carbs 3, protein 5

Cranberries and Cauliflower Rice Pudding

Prep time: 5 minutes | Cooking time: 20 minutes | Servings: 6

Ingredients:

- 1 cup cauliflower rice
- 2 cups almond milk
- ½ cup cranberries
- 1 teaspoon vanilla extract

Directions:

In a pan that fits your air fryer, mix all the ingredients, whisk a bit, put the pan in the fryer and cook at 360 degrees F for 20 minutes. Stir the pudding, divide into bowls and serve cold.

Nutrition: calories 211, fat 5, fiber 2, carbs 4, protein 7

Lemon Cookies

Prep time: 10 minutes | Cooking time: 20 minutes | Servings: 12

Ingredients:

- 1 cup coconut cream
- ¼ cup cashew butter, soft
- ¼ cup swerve
- 1 egg, whisked
- Juice of 1 lemon
- 1 teaspoon lemon peel, grated
- 1 teaspoon baking powder

Directions:

In a bowl, combine all the ingredients gradually and stir well. Spoon balls this on a cookie sheet lined with parchment paper and flatten them. Put the cookie sheet in the fryer and cook at 350 degrees F for 20 minutes. Serve the cookies cold.

Nutrition: calories 121, fat 5, fiber 1, carbs 4, protein 2

Mini Lava Cakes
Prep time: 10 minutes | Cooking time: 20 minutes | Servings: 4

Ingredients:
- 3 ounces dark chocolate, melted
- ¼ cup coconut oil, melted
- 2 tablespoons swerve
- 2 eggs, whisked
- ¼ teaspoon vanilla extract
- 1 tablespoon almond flour
- Cooking spray

Directions:

In bowl, combine all the ingredients except the cooking spray and whisk really well. Divide this into 4 ramekins greased with cooking spray, put them in the fryer and cook at 360 degrees F for 20 minutes. Serve warm.

Nutrition: calories 161, fat 12, fiber 1, carbs 4, protein 7

Espresso Cookies
Prep time: 5 minutes | Cooking time: 15 minutes | Servings: 12

Ingredients:
- 8 tablespoons ghee, melted
- 1 cup almond flour
- ¼ cup brewed espresso
- ¼ cup swerve
- ½ tablespoon cinnamon powder
- 2 teaspoons baking powder
- 2 eggs, whisked

Directions:

In a bowl, mix all the ingredients and whisk well. Spread medium balls on a cookie sheet lined parchment paper, flatten them, put the cookie sheet in your air fryer and cook at 350 degrees F for 15 minutes. Serve the cookies cold.

Nutrition: calories 134, fat 12, fiber 2, carbs 4, protein 2

Sponge Ricotta Cake
Prep time: 5 minutes | *Cooking time:* 30 minutes | *Servings:* 8

Ingredients:
- 1 cup ricotta, soft
- 1/3 swerve
- 3 eggs, whisked
- 1 cup almond flour
- 7 tablespoons ghee, melted
- 1 teaspoon baking powder
- Cooking spray

Directions:
In a bowl, combine all the ingredients except the cooking spray and stir them very well. Grease a cake pan that fits the air fryer with the cooking spray and pour the cake mix inside. Put the pan in the fryer and cook at 350 degrees F for 30 minutes. Cool the cake down, slice and serve.

Nutrition: calories 210, fat 12, fiber 3, carbs 6, protein 9

Chocolate Strawberry Cups
Prep time: 5 minutes | *Cooking time:* 10 minutes | *Servings:* 8

Ingredients:
- 16 strawberries, halved
- 2 tablespoons coconut oil
- 2 cups chocolate chips, melted

Directions:
In a pan that fits your air fryer, mix the strawberries with the oil and the melted chocolate chips, toss gently, put the pan in the air fryer and cook at 340 degrees F for 10 minutes. Divide into cups and serve cold.

Nutrition: calories 162, fat 5, fiber 3, carbs 5, protein 6

Recipe Index

Cashew Pork Mix, 193

COCONUT FLAKES
Chicken Cubes, 99
Crispy Salmon Fillets, 128
Crispy Chicken Tenders, 161
Crusted Lamb Cutlets, 208
Coconut Bars, 240
Avocado Granola, 256

COCONUT FLOUR
Rosemary Mushroom Balls, 101
Shrimp Balls, 104
Almond Cupcakes, 239
Coconut Donuts, 242
Raspberry Muffins, 244
Cream Cheese Brownies, 247
Yogurt Cake, 250
Strawberry Cake, 254

COCONUT MILK
Cheesy Spinach Muffins, 22
Coconut Cauliflower Pudding, 31
Blackberries Bowls, 40
Strawberries Oatmeal, 41
Coconut Cauliflower Risotto, 82
Broccoli Dip, 119
Turkey and Cheese Balls, 122
Coconut and Chili Pork, 187
Kale and Mushrooms Mix, 223
Coconut Donuts, 242
Cocoa Cake, 245
Spiced Avocado Pudding, 254
Cauliflower Rice and Plum Pudding, 255

COURGETTES
Courgettes Casserole, 63
Duck Breast and Veggies, 178

CRANBERRIES
Cranberries and Cauliflower Rice Pudding, 257

CREAM CHEESE
Creamy Almond and Cheese Mix, 16
Turkey and Zucchini Casserole, 51
Mini Peppers Mix, 73
Cream Cheese Zucchini, 90
Salmon Spread, 109
Tomatoes Dip, 120
Peppers and Cheese Dip, 121
Mustard Pork Chops, 185
Cream Cheese Brownies, 247
Cream and Coconut Cups, 248
Cream Cheese and Zucchinis Bars, 248
Chocolate Pudding, 250
Strawberry Cake, 254

CUCUMBERS
Cucumber Salsa, 117
Chili Lamb and Cucumber Salsa, 207

CURRANTS
Currant Cream, 256
Currant Pudding, 256
Currant Cookies, 257

DUCK
Duck and Mushroom Rice, 174
Duck Breast and Blackberry Sauce, 174
Spiced Duck Legs, 175
Thyme Duck Legs, 175
Cinnamon Duck Breasts, 176
Cardamom Duck Legs, 176
Duck with Cinnamon and Olives, 177
Vanilla Duck Legs, 177
Duck Breast and Veggies, 178
Duck Breast and Pepper Sauce, 178
Duck and Eggplant Mix, 179
Creamy Duck Mix, 179
Duck, Peppers and Asparagus Mix, 180
Duck Salad, 180
Duck Breast and Cranberry Sauce, 181
Parsley Duck Breast Mix, 181

Conclusion

The Ketogenic air fryer recipes collection you've just discovered is probably one of the best cooking guides available these days. All the recipes are so easy to make in the comfort of your own home and they all follow the Ketogenic principles.

On one hand, you probably know by now that cooking with an air fryer is really the latest innovation in cooking. Air fryers are so popular due to their many advantages. These modern kitchen appliances allow you to cook perfect meals with minimum effort. All the dishes made with an air fryer require little time and cooking skills.

On the other hand, the Ketogenic diet has shown its multiple benefits to so many people. This diet can change your metabolism and can improve your appearance.

The cooking journal brought to you today combines cooking in an air fryer with the richness of Ketogenic recipes.

Cooking Ketogenic dishes in an air fryer can be so easy and fun. So, don't hesitate! Get this recipes collection and start cooking some healthy, rich and textured meals using just one modern appliance: the air fryer!

CPSIA information can be obtained
at www.ICGtesting.com
Printed in the USA
LVHW090156160120
643819LV00001B/45